CHRONICALLY
unstoppable

HOW MY LIFE WENT FROM
FIGHT-OR-FLIGHT TO *FREE*

AUDREY MARIE

Chronically Unstoppable: How My Life Went from Fight-or-Flight to Free
Copyright © 2024 Audrey Marie
Cover art by Danielle Ballard

World Publishing and Productions
PO Box 8722, Jupiter, FL 33468
worldpublishingandproductions.com

All rights reserved. This book is protected under the copyright laws of the United States of America. No portion of this book may be reproduced, distributed, or transmitted in any form, including photocopying, recording, or other electronic or mechanical methods, without the written permission of the publisher, excepted in the case of brief quotations embodied in reviews or certain other non-commercial uses permitted by copyright law.

ISBN: 978-1-957111-24-7
Library of Congress Control Number: 2024901334

This book is dedicated to my mom.

*I wouldn't be here without you, and I am beyond grateful to have you fighting alongside me.
I could do it because I AM exactly like you.*

Contents

Nice to Meet You	IX
Introduction	XIII
The Diagnoses	XVII
PART ONE: LIVING CAREFREE	1
1. The Not-So-Nuclear Family	3
2. Building Blocks of Faith	6
3. Listen to Mom	9
4. "Career-Ending/Beginning" Injury	14
5. The Perfect Storm	19
PART TWO: LIFE-LASTING MOMENTS	27
6. And the Process Begins...	29
7. Take My Problem and Double It	34
8. No Explanations	37
9. Not That Bad	41
10. Calm Before the Storm	45

11.	Brain-Changing Trauma	52
12.	Here We Go Again (Just Successful)	58
13.	Fire Ignited	62
14.	Complex Regional Pain Syndrome	70
15.	My Pain is Related to What?	76
16.	Knock Back—Let Fly	83
17.	To Keep or Not to Keep Faith	87
18.	Stagnant Suffering	92
19.	Just Let Me Drive	98
20.	Rilee	102
21.	Show Me I Can Do It	107
22.	Rally Around Me	111
PART THREE: FINDING HOPE		117
Disclaimer		118
23.	Waking Nightmare	119
24.	We All Need Support	129
25.	Am I Behind?	138
26.	One Last Shot	144
27.	Virtual Treatment	151
28.	Finding Him	167
29.	Non-Representative Insurance	179

30.	The Fight of My Life	183
31.	No Embarrassment with Amena	192
32.	Exciting, Difficult Farewell	196
33.	Same Life, Different Me	204
PART FOUR: EVERYTHING CLICKS		209
34.	Right Where I Should Be	211
35.	No Matter What, A Win is a Win	217
36.	Welcome Home	232
37.	Catching Up?	237
38.	24/7 Guards	243
39.	Driver's Seat	246
40.	A Letter from Me to You	252

Nice to Meet You

What is the worst pain you've ever experienced? Now, what if I told you that pain would never go away for the rest of your life? Would you choose to continue truly living, or would you get into bed with the hope that the pain will somehow stop?

By the time I was 17, this hypothetical scenario became my reality. You see, new friend, my life has been everything but boring. Currently, I am simply trying to figure my future out. You know, everyone's favorite point in their life—when you get pressured into getting a job and getting married even though you are not even a quarter of the way through with your life. This is one of the first "typical" experiences I have had in life because, honestly, I've struggled in the normal category.

I know, I know, "normal" is not a well-liked word in the English language, so in other words, I have not had the opportunity to be a part of the typical paths people take as they get older.

AUDREY MARIE

What do you do when you don't have a choice but to fall behind in life? It took me seven years to find the answer to this. But that is why I am writing this book. I want to speed up those seven years for you. You will figure all of that out when you read this book. I can't get into it all yet, or I might scare you away, so instead, I am just going to introduce myself.

My name is Audrey, and as I said, I am a 23-year-old young adult (I'm still not comfortable with saying "woman"). I graduated in 2021 from college with a major in political science and a minor in security and conflict studies. I work for an anti-trafficking organization called The National Trafficking Sheltered Alliance. Oh, I'm also getting my masters in homeland security and emergency preparedness.

As you can see, I am incredibly active. But that has only happened within the past year. If you would have spoken to me prior to 2021, you would not even recognize me now. The only part of me that has stayed consistent is my persistence and courage. No matter what, I don't give up. But today, I can say I have a wise outlook on life. I strongly believe anyone with a condition develops the same thing.

I know what you are probably thinking, "That's great, Audrey, but why are you writing a book?" Well, person who bothered to pick this book up, I have a story that will shock you. A story that has made me into the person I am today. I wonder how many people can pinpoint the moment their life changed. I know I sure can.

I have a condition called Complex Regional Pain Syndrome. In a few short pages, you will read an explanation of all my conditions. Here, I will just be very vague. CRPS is known to most as the worst pain known to man. Its cause is unknown, but typically, it comes after a trauma of some sort. Many people don't know about it because it is somewhat rare. In shortened terms, CRPS happens to those who have their brain malfunction, just like any electronic device of your choice. Only I can't turn myself off and fully restart. The malfunction can last forever. Yes, forever. What a difficult concept.

So, am I writing this book because I am cured? Sadly, I have to say absolutely not. I still battle my conditions every single day. Once you have chronic pain, you tend to become numb to it. It's there, but it's just part of your life. In my words, it is what it is. But that doesn't mean good things haven't come from the conditions. I can say I've met more incredible people than I can count. I am at a job I never thought I would be capable of. I have a slight following on social media. I got a dog I will never forget, and I have one who is now my best friend. And I am also closer with God. When I thought all was dark, I realized He was there, watching me behind the shadows. Ready to catch me when I fall.

Not only all of this, but I am also living in the center of a city—in an incredible apartment. It still shocks me. Almost a waking dream. Just by reading this one paragraph, you'd think I now have the most perfect life. That even if I "claim" to have a chronic pain condition, I'm living a life that shows I am perfectly fine: young, living in a city, continuing school, and working a job—the whole package.

Sure, my life is great now. I've learned a lot about managing my pain and stress. But I had a hard time for a while. That may be an understatement. I was absolutely miserable and not functioning. Don't worry, you'll soon understand. I want you to walk away with the feeling that anything is possible. Yes, bad things happen, but that doesn't mean you can't have a happy and incredible life. But for now, kick your feet up, get comfy, and be prepared to experience the worst part of my life—

Introduction

We all learn at a young age to visit the doctor when we feel unwell. We arrive at the appointment optimistic that we will leave with hope in the form of medicine or a treatment recommendation. But all too often, our doctor's visit ends with the disappointing statement, "If it doesn't feel better in 14 days, come back." Although that isn't exactly what we wanted, having a timeframe can still offer peace.

But what do you do when you aren't offered medicine, a promising treatment, or even a timeframe? How do you handle it when you are told your condition could last forever?

Chronic conditions can derail our life. They can rip us down to our bare bones and eventually take away our humanity. Sadly, I learned this all too early in life. Perhaps you picked this book up because you or a loved one are dealing with a chronic condition, or maybe you are just interested in my story. No matter the reason, I am happy to say you are at the right place.

This book will give you a complete view of my life—a life riddled with chronic pain. I hope my candor about the processing I went through that ultimately brought me to a place of peace with my condition will help you with whatever life has thrown at you. I'm not a psychologist, nor do I have a degree in the science of pain, but I have the highest expertise there truly is—learning to live a full life despite the constant attack of pain.

My battle was not easy, as you will read. I have divided my journey into four different parts that tell the story: 1) Living in ignorant bliss. 2) The unexpected bursting of flames. 3) Losing and finding hope. 4) Truly living.

In these pages, I chronicle how I held, lost, and then found hope again. Although my desire is that you think about your own story as you read mine, I hope it won't cause you to dwell on hardships or the things you may have missed out on. Instead, I want this book to offer you validation. Validation of everything you have gone through.

To show you, dear reader, that every reaction, interaction, condition, and behavior is reasonable, I take you into my life's deepest and most intimate points. When I was much younger and beginning to experience this illness I couldn't begin to understand, I desperately wanted to find someone who had made it out or even on the other side of chronic pain. But no matter how many times I tried, I failed. I wrote this book to ensure that nothing like that would ever happen again.

Whether you are reading my story out of interest, for inspiration, or as a last effort to find someone who understands what you are going through, this book is for you. And I am happy you picked it up.

I do ask you to please read this book with an open mind. In it, I offer many recommendations for handling your health, but it is more than a book full of recommendations—it is a story of my growth that I pray will help you on your journey. So, even if you are tired and feeling ready to give in, I ask you for your willingness to listen to my story as you process yours. Who knows, you might find that something I have experienced resonates with you beyond belief.

As you turn each page, watch how my mindset has evolved. Treat this book as your closest friend and the key that will open up an understanding for you. Flip this page and begin the journey—a journey that may feel achingly familiar to you yet refreshingly hopeful.

The Diagnoses

I would like to make something clear. In this chapter, I will be discussing three different conditions that I have been diagnosed with during the past five years. I will define these diseases in my own words. Personally, I find it is easier to understand an illness when I hear it described in layperson's terms rather than in words from a scientific study or a doctor's perspective—so that is how I am laying it out for you. However, if you want to understand the intricacies of these diseases further, including precise statistics and up-to-date data and findings, please feel free to do your own research. My goal is to explain what I have experienced in a way that will help you understand what it is like to live with these diseases and how they *really* affect an individual's life.

Complex Regional Pain Syndrome (CRPS)

Well, well, well. Here I am—doing the thing I never wanted to do: defining Complex Regional Pain Syndrome.

Those four words controlled my life for far too long. I denied them, ignored them, and spent time wondering what they *actually* mean.

It took me five long, excruciating years to finally get a grip on the disease, and I will attempt to explain it to you in my own words. This is a bit tricky as I don't know if you even have a connection to CRPS, but that's part of the problem. People without an attachment to any disease don't often feel a need or motivation to take the time to understand what someone else may be experiencing.

Believe me, I get it. Life is full of intricate diseases, ailments, and issues. Thank goodness we all don't have to deal with all of them! But I want to encourage you to grow in empathy. I wrote this book, in part, so that you, the reader, will gain a wider perspective on some of the hidden ailments people around you may be dealing with. The more you understand this particular disease, the more you will appreciate this book and my perspective.

Complex Regional Pain Syndrome, or CRPS, is a neurological disorder that occurs between the brain and the body's pain receptors. Allow me to simplify the complexity of the condition because that has been the best way for me to understand it. Typically, the condition begins after an injury to the body, which causes the brain to send pain signals to a particular limb, which then becomes affected. For most people, pain signals are critical for human survival. Sadly, for people like me, those pain signals begin never-ending torture.

Pain signals in average people follow a "normal" pattern with which you are likely familiar. First, the person feels pain; then, the body reacts with a biological process. This can include many different symptoms: swelling, changing color, becoming immensely painful, or limiting usability, for example. Once the injury has healed, the brain stops sending those signals, and the body returns to normal. Makes sense, right?

My body is different. Let's say someone with CRPS gets an injury. Their brain sends a pain signal, and the person reacts as anyone else would: using ice compresses, easing up on doing activities that cause pain, etc. But then CRPS comes in, causing the person's brain to get stuck in the pain cycle. The brain constantly sends pain signals because it feels like there is an ongoing injury. Even if the actual injury is completely healed, the brain continues to see the injury and feel the pain, telling the nervous system that there is an injury or threat to the body even though there isn't one. This causes immense and ongoing pain to a limb, limbs, or even the whole body. Meanwhile, medical tests do not reveal any "proof" that the pain even exists.

This cycle is horrific to those few people in the world who suffer from the condition. It causes intense burning and an unimaginable deep, deep ache. The body of the affected individual shows physical symptoms, too. These symptoms can be anything from swelling to sweat to even actual burns.

I often explain CRPS pain like this: Imagine your limb (or whatever affected area) is on fire. Then, on top of the surface fire, a deep pain—an indescribable pressure and ache—extends down into the bone. This type of burning can be conceptualized by envisioning the pain from the worst sunburn and multiplying it by a million. You know, that sunburn that keeps you up at night? Well, CRPS makes that look easy. This, along with typical nerve pain, is what is responsible for the CRPS hell.

I apologize if this is hard to read. Trust me, I don't like writing it, let alone living it. This type of pain stays for years at a dysfunctional level. Someone suffering from this would do anything and everything to stop or lessen the pain. No matter *what* or *who* they lose.

And, to top it off, although medical tests are useful to rule out other conditions, there is no medical test that can diagnose CRPS. This fact plays a part in the insecurities of those suffering from the disease. The person struggles to come to terms with having to have faith in their medical professionals while never receiving validation on paper.

Post-Traumatic Stress Disorder (PTSD)

PTSD is, overall, widely understood by the population—but it is not a disease limited to veterans or victims of violence or sexual assault. Due to this misconception, I never would have said I could have PTSD because nothing *bad* has ever happened to me. But I was so wrong. I will explain it in a way that shows you how it presents itself in me.

My PTSD stems from medical trauma (you will learn about it in future chapters). After that trauma occurred, I had many reactions throughout each day. A single word could separate me from my life and force me into an out-of-body experience. My heart would begin to race. I stopped being able to control my thoughts and memories my mind would go to. Showers were as scary to me as a criminal with a gun.

PTSD has me on high alert all day, every day. I am consistently checking for dangers without even realizing it. In the blink of an eye, it pulls me out of the present. Suddenly, I am back to when my trauma occurred. I even feel the sensations I experienced on that very day. It takes a while for anyone to pull me back. PTSD is the condition that reminds you of the worst day of your life.

Functional Neurological Symptom Disorder (FNSD)

I want to preface this by cautioning you against reading randomly about any condition you are diagnosed with; instead, let your medical team explain it to you. I made that mistake when I was first diagnosed with FNSD. And let me tell you, I was furious at my team (yes, the team that ended up saving my life. But it was rocky for a while there). My FNSD occurred a few months after I was diagnosed with CRPS, and it got worse with time. But, it wasn't diagnosed for four years.

Let me explain this condition to you the way I understand it. Functional Neurological System Disorder is a condition in which your nervous system doesn't function correctly under stress. This usually occurs after a traumatic event (like surgery and never-ending pain).

Here is how it happens. A trauma basically snaps the brain into an atypical response. That means it avoids the usual pathway and creates a new one—so when there is a stress reactor, the brain uses the new FNSD pathway. This rerouting can be traumatic to the brain. When the stress goes through the new pathway, it presents in other ways, leading to many possible symptoms, such as tremors (me), stuttering (me), blanking out or freezing (me), seizures, paralysis, loss of balance (me), and so much more.

The longer the brain uses this new pathway, the harder it is for it to return to using the original pathway. As time passes, the entire nervous system—including breathing, heart rate, blood pressure, and sweat—begins to alter how it functions in response to stress. Every time the person encounters stress—whether traumatic or not—the nervous system reacts in atypical ways. However, if the trauma continues throughout time, like in other chronic pain patients, the path begins to become more and more cleared. My neuropsychologist explained it as "a road in the snow." She said the more cars drive down a road in the snow, the more the road becomes cleared and stays clear. So, you can think of it like this: the main road in the brain of a person with FNSD was plowed; the side street has to be completely cleared.

PART ONE
living carefree

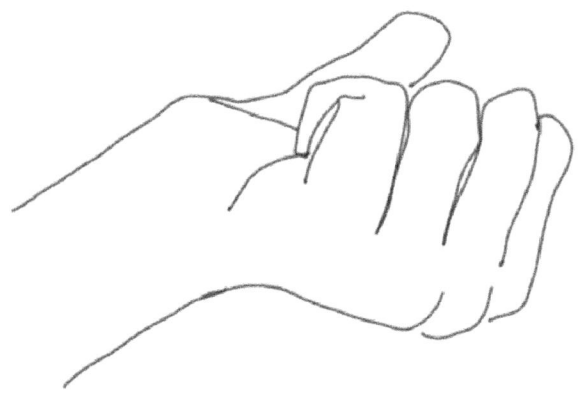

Chapter 1

The Not-So-Nuclear Family

I was born into a very basic family. At the time, I had one older sister, a mom, and a dad. Everything a little kid could wish for. My parents had just built a house in a small town in Virginia. Not only this, my grandparents on my mom's side (whom we are very close with) owned a condo right on the beach in North Myrtle Beach. Apparently, my infant self wasn't a fan, but that changed quickly.

I was told I was a funny baby/toddler. When I was four and about to go to kindergarten, my mom decided to ask me a few questions. You know, as parents do to make sure their kid shows they are a good parent. She would ask me to say the alphabet.

"A-B-C-D-E-X-Y-Z-Q-P-T."

That would always be my immediate response. My mom recalled being a little concerned at this point. So, she tried another question.

"Push the right shapes through the box with their matching slots."

Me, being me, would sit for twenty minutes slamming a triangle into the circle slot, knowing it was the wrong shape.

"I don't know what she knows. I think she could be a little off," my mom told the kindergarten teacher. It was quite the change for my mother from my older sister. Let's just say Emily was quite the "perfect child" (as a firstborn typically is).

The teacher had class with me and spoke with my mom again afterward.

"She knows it all. She is ahead of others. ABC's, shapes, all of it."

My mom was in complete shock. But that is just my personality. I'm a jokester. I like for life to be exciting. I also don't want to be basic or average. Even my 4-year-old self knew that. Remember this for the rest of the book. I most certainly wasn't average. Not only this, I also had a sense of humor. It was always difficult for me to take things too seriously. Anything that I deemed 'boring,' I loved to spice up. It's who I have always been, even to this very day.

Within the blink of an eye, our small family turned into five kids and one adult: me, my older sister, the twins (boy and girl), and a younger sister. I know you are wondering, one adult? Well, my father was not as dedicated to the family as everyone else. He started wreaking havoc when I was eight, and then finally left the house (and my life) for good when I was headed to high school. Let's just say he didn't go quietly. He and his alcohol made sure to leave an everlasting effect on the family. But no matter what, we stayed strong. We did what we had to do. As simple as that.

• • • • ● • ● • • •

I know life can be hard, my friend. It throws us curveballs. Some can be fun and exciting, while others may be incredibly hard. Both, however, change the trajectory of our lives.

I know the experience with my father was detrimental to the entire family. It was painful and terrifying. My life would look different if he had stayed in our lives. Or even if he had left in a less disruptive way. However, humans are extremely adaptive. You do what you have to do in order to survive. It's easy to look back and wonder what could've been if a single event had gone differently. But I wholeheartedly believe that the events from my father prepared me for what was to come. Want to know why? It taught my family and me to never quit and to be there for each other no matter what.

Chapter 2

Building Blocks of Faith

My mom raised us all with faith in the home.

We were taught to go to church every weekend and on every major holiday. We did CCD (school for church) and made sure to do things for the church community. But overall, that was about it with our extent of faith. I never read the full Bible, and I didn't have many personal conversations with God. We were taught to love Him and be grateful for Him.

We went through phases of saying a prayer before every meal or before bed, but it never seemed to fully stick. I was always confident God was there, but there were times when I would wonder and question. My mom happily welcomed questions if they were simply curiosity. There were, of course, some things my mom was strict about with faith. I remember her always saying, "Don't say God's name in vain." And she would ensure we didn't talk during church. I'd like to say we were average in the level we practiced faith.

CHRONICALLY UNSTOPPABLE

Even growing up without a father, my faith was strong. There was never a question or concern about God's existence. My mom was so strong during this time and taught us that God is with us no matter what. We found peace in going to church. It was somewhere that my father wasn't. I was able to sit with the family and not stress or worry about him walking in. It was a constant I could count on every week.

When my father was terrorizing the house, he would make me feel a lot of horrific emotions. My biggest focus, however, was making sure I could protect my family. Us against him. Night after night, he'd get drunk and prove that he had no care for me.

"If you loved me, you wouldn't leave"—walks out the door.

"Please just stop already"—looks at me in the face and gets louder.

There was nothing we could do. A tyrant was living in our home.

But did I ever get angry with God? No.

Did I ever question all God could do? Absolutely not.

Did I think I was being punished? Nope.

That's because my father was an outside force. If God had control over humans' actions, we wouldn't have murderers, rapists, arsonists, you name it. I didn't feel the need to blame Him for something someone else did. We as humans want so badly to find someone to blame in order to make sense of what has happened to us. I didn't need to blame my faith because I already had a tangible person to blame. You may wonder how I understood how this could happen when I fully trusted my faith. Well, my incredible mother could answer that question easily.

"God gives everyone a cross to bear; everything from dad is ours," my mom explained.

I latched onto that idea. My faith would never waiver. Well, that's what I thought.

• • • • ● • ● • • •

Friend, you tell me: What if we are given multiple crosses to bear? Do we keep faith? You'll soon see I didn't. Take it from me: you don't realize you had that level of faith until it is slowly ripped away. Pried out of my hands without giving me anything else to hold onto. CRPS wasn't an outside force. It was inside. And it stole the thing most constant: God.

Chapter 3

Listen to Mom

I was 4 when my twin siblings were born. One—Olivia—was a girl, and the other—Robert—was a boy. As you can assume by how I was as a child, I was obsessed with the boy. As we got older, I realized he didn't have a father around—meaning no male figure. I began to learn how to play every sport, do boy's hair, tie a tie, you name it. This way, I would be able to stand in the gap for him every time he needed it. We became incredibly close. We still are to this day. It didn't matter that I felt the need to learn all the sports because I never fit into the gender stereotypes that come with being a little girl. I used to throw fits when I had to put a dress on or wear shoes that were anything other than flip-flops or tennis shoes.

When I was in preschool, my mom put me in ballet class. My older sister was a dancer, and that's usually a go-to for parents—so my mom thought, why not? I walked into ballet with my tights and leotard, started class, and ran out crying within the first 10 minutes. Saying I hated it was an understatement. It just shows that we are all made different. That doesn't mean one way is better than the other. There was no judgment from my mom; I will be forever grateful for that.

After the failed dance class, my mom put me in soccer. I loved everything about the sport. Of course, it was a small recreational team in our town, but it didn't matter. I was ready to be on the field at any moment. Between that, recess at school, and helping my mom around the house, I never really sat still. It was obvious that being busy was my way of handling the stress that my father caused. Avoiding what was going on in life was my main coping mechanism. Make sure to note the word avoidance. It will come into play quite a bit when I am at the age of 16.

This non-girly trend continued as I went into elementary school. Girls would go to recess and walk around and talk or play on the monkey bars. I was the one playing basketball with all the boys on the blacktop. As I look back, I can tell I was a tough cookie. Those boys in school would push me over, and it didn't bother me. We even tried to play tackle football (but, of course, got in trouble). I felt more comfortable being super active; it allowed me to blow off steam. Even back then, I thought there was too much drama with girls. Guys were very simple. And to be completely honest, I just loved sports.

By the time I was in 5th grade, I had my first broken bone. I know, I know, you may be thinking that is a little too early for a broken bone. Curious as to how? Well, being the tough kid I was, I grew an interest in skateboarding. That interest sparked when I watched a show, "Zeke and Luther," with my little brother. After talking it over with my mom, I got my very first skateboard. My excitement could not be contained. The day I got it, right after school, I ran into the house and begged my mom to let me go ride it in our garage. After a ten-minute argument, she agreed—just in the garage until dinner was ready.

I grabbed my shoes, put on my helmet, and ran outside. I set the skateboard on the ground and jumped right on it. I rode from one side of the garage to the other with my hands held out sideways. That was enough for my 9-year-old self to determine I could probably do a trick.

I've seen an ollie on the show. I bet I can do it.

I wasn't supposed to do any tricks, but let's not forget, I always liked to surprise people, and I always wanted life to be exciting. At least my version of exciting. So, naturally, I had to do a quick trick before my mom came out.

I set the skateboard up, got onto it, put my hands out and...BAM!

AUDREY MARIE

I fell backward in a blink of an eye. I let out the biggest yell, and my mom came running out.

"I hit my elbow. Mom, I can't move my elbow."

I was crying more than I had ever cried before. Although my mom wasn't happy with me, she didn't yell at me. Instead, she quickly said I needed to go to the E.R. As much as I didn't want to, I had a feeling my elbow was in rough shape.

• • • • ● • ● • • •

I want to point something out to you, friend. This was my first moment of intense pain that I can recall. Sure, pain is relative. What could be the worst to you might not be the worst to me. But this incident required me to be physically strong. I had been mentally strong by this point, but physical is a whole other battle. However, this taught me to make the best of what we are given. Not only that, but there is no way to prepare for life. Oh, plus, always listen to your parents.

• • • ● • ● • • •

A few hours and waiting room snacks later, I had a wrap around my entire elbow. Turns out, I broke my growth plate in my elbow. Lovely. Don't worry, a few months later, the giant, heavy cast was off, and I was back to my active self. Overall, I was durable and didn't let anything get me down for long. This came in great use later in life. It's amazing how life skills come to us early on. Maybe it is a way of God preparing us for the worst and hoping for the best?

Chapter 4

"Career-Ending/Beginning" Injury

By the time I was in middle school, my youngest sibling, Gia, came along. I had played soccer for several years. It was kind of my sport. Something that made me feel confident, but also let me blow off steam. I was a stressed-out kid since my father left the family (again, not quietly). Soccer allowed me to focus on something aside from that for a few hours a week.

I got pretty good at the sport! Defense was often my position. If I'm being totally honest, I was phenomenal at defending. That ball would cross over the half-field line, and I was on it.

As I got older, I would play both defense and offense. Sure, I was fast, but I was also fearless. It didn't matter how big the boys were or how willing they were to truck me over; I would protect that goal. An amazing trait to have as a young girl. I quickly became well-known around the league. My favorite reaction was when guys were talking about how mad they were that I was on the field. Kind of hilarious.

I was a freshman in high school when I got my third concussion. Heading other players' heads was a common theme for me. Man, did the concussions hurt. And they would make me miss school. In the plainest of terms, this was NOT GOOD. Being 14 and experiencing concussions can cause a lot of issues. However, I continued to play. I wasn't going to quit; it was my love.

During the first half of my 9th-grade year, I was conditioning for the school's soccer team every day after school. I was scared at first. I had so much self-doubt that everyone would be better, but I can't put into words how much I loved it. This was my first team with all girls, and I was not complaining! I was in the best shape I had ever been, and I was learning so much. Not all the nicest people were a part of it, but it was still my dream.

In November, my mom promised that if I made the spring team, she would buy me custom cleats from Nike! I always wanted a pair, and I knew I was getting so close! In order to continue improving my skills, I joined the school's scrimmage indoor league for the winter. Then, I had my second life-changing event:

I broke my foot on the very first day of winter scrimmage.

It happened pretty suddenly. I went to shoot the ball, and a girl came behind and stepped on my foot. It cracked, and I felt quite a bit of pain. Sadly, thinking back, the pain wasn't that bad. But for a "normal" system the pain was bad. Believe it or not, I played the rest of the game (although I cried the whole time). This is another representation of my strength and courage to keep moving forward. I had just broken my ankle but remained on the field. Even though it hurt, I felt the need to continue. I wanted to.

But this break made me rethink everything. I was 15 and already had three concussions and now a bad ankle break. Was this my life plan? Did I want to play soccer for my future?

Is it all worth it?

What a question.

• • • ● • ● • • •

Sure, this was the first time this question came into my life. But without a doubt, it wouldn't be the last.

Any decision regarding whether something is worth it can drive someone mad. Unfortunately, we can't see into the future, so how willing are we to risk our health for an activity? Some of you may say you will risk it all. You may feel as if it were the only thing you would ever be good at. I will say I felt like that for a long time. Although I had guitar lessons, I still felt that nothing came as naturally as soccer.

However, as we get older, we start to see different points of view. My main question for myself was, what do I want to do with my future? Is it related to soccer? If you are or have experienced these feelings, then you are not alone. It is okay to ask questions when you don't know what the future will hold. I know my future turned out completely different than I thought.

· · · · • · • • · ·

I stopped going to conditioning when I was in a cast. That meant it was hard to find things to look forward to in school. Well, rather quickly, God did me a favor and put me in theater class as one of my electives. It was a class I shockingly loved.

I was never someone to perform, but I was putting so much energy into every class. Meanwhile, I was also in a tech theater elective. This was a class about creating all the set design pieces of theater. I have a friend who always tells me things happen for a reason. Ending up in theater showed me just how many other talents I had. No matter what we are feeling, God always has a plan. Learning to trust that plan is the difficult part.

AUDREY MARIE

I quickly realized I loved theater just as much as I loved soccer. But have I ever gotten injured doing theater? Not at that point. I mean, how could a non-physical activity harm me? It's not like soccer, where I could get a concussion from deliberate movement. Ha! Who would've thought? Maybe this was when my desire to try new things stopped. My one activity (soccer) stopped due to injury. The next activity (theater) would stop a short three years later due to horrific injury.

Would I go back and stay with soccer if I could? I wouldn't change a thing. I know, I know, cliché. But trust me, you'll end up understanding.

Chapter 5

The Perfect Storm

When I was younger, I was always afraid of doctors and needles. I was the kid screaming in the pediatrician's office as if the doctor was holding a gun instead of a needle. I will be honest and say I needed to toughen up a little bit. Ok. A lot. But I was just a kid. An innocent kid who didn't have a routine of receiving shots or other medical treatments.

• • • ● ● • ● • • •

Sometimes, it's nice not to be entirely "tough" as a kid. Kids should have the opportunity to grow and experience life without living in fear. At what point in someone's life should they stop being scared of shots? Do we as a society agree on an age? Honestly, I believe it should come naturally. We shouldn't decide a set time that things should get easier. We don't know what people have gone through to make them have specific reactions.

Sometimes, dear friend, the ones who appear strongest have suffered the most. I can say I wasn't given the choice of when I would be less fearful of doctors. I wasn't ready for my future. But nothing could have prepared me for the summer when everything changed.

• • • • • • • • • •

My sophomore year of high school was one of the best years of my life. Like I said in the last chapter, I had made the decision to switch from soccer to theater. I started out doing lights for the competition play. Not only did I create the light looks, but I also ran them during the show. I remember going away to Norfolk, Virginia (my first overnight travel trip) to do the first statewide competition. When the show was over, our group went backstage, and they all started clapping for me.

"Audrey that lighting system was so difficult, way to go."

"This performance was owed to Audrey."

I fell in love with the environment, the art, the people, everything. I knew that theater, acting, this overall art, was my calling. It didn't take long before I took to the stage and started acting. My very first show was *Charlotte's Web*. I was one of the village people. I know, I know, the star of the show *sarcasm*. But I fell in love with acting even more. I loved the rush you got before going on stage and the fact that you still end up sweating. I used to believe sweating meant that you were giving it 100% of yourself. In other words, it was something I WANTED to happen. Sweat now has a negative connotation in my mind.

I felt like I was on top of the world my whole sophomore year. My verbally abusive father had finally left the house and officially moved out of our lives, and I had found a group of friends I loved. I quickly became close with them and was finally feeling more confident in myself. Soccer had always been my focus and goal, until I experienced the environment of theater. I began to take acting classes and I was more involved in the department at my school. Things were finally looking up!

Even my stress and protective instinct (forced upon me by my father) was down. Life was coming together. I actually felt *normal*. However, here I'd like to point out that normal has no exact definition. It looks different for every person. The image of what I thought was normal was pretty simple. Being normal was someone who didn't have to live in fear from one of their parents. I was at the point in my life where I was able to relax. Breathe. Although it didn't last very long, I was living in pure bliss.

This acting path led me to a somewhat significant role in the spring musical *Into the Woods*. I got the role of Jack's Mother. I didn't practice this role. I didn't even audition for it. I felt like it wasn't my place as a sophomore to audition for a higher-up role. I actually auditioned for the granny who came on the stage maybe five times and had very few lines. I remember asking one of the top actors in the department, Elise, to help me with the audition. She even came over to my house, we sang through the audition piece, and I practiced the granny. Honestly, it was a blast of a night.

After I finished the granny audition, my theater director called me into the audience where he always sat.

"Go up and do Jack's Mother with Andre," said Mr. D.

I was terrified, but I had been friends with Andre for a while, so I felt comfortable. I went on stage, did the scene, and people were dying from laughing so hard (yes, the character was for comedic relief). Between the character types and Andre and I's relationship outside of theater, the scene seemed to work. I found out that night that I got the role!

When the show opened, I remember people being shocked that I was able to sing and that I could act out the role of the obnoxious mother. I loved the play, the experience, the design, and my role more than anything. The only downside? The costume. That costume was layered more than I could count. We would have to put it on at the start of every dress rehearsal and show and wear it for at least five hours. Then, by intermission of every show, I switched to an even heavier costume WITH gloves! I would sweat buckets every time we would rehearse or perform. But honestly, I kind of loved it. It felt like a workout combined with acting. It gave me the same exhausted feeling I loved from soccer.

In Virginia, it usually becomes warmer in the spring. Not only this, but there was so much moving onstage and incredibly hot lights. Here was the equation for the complete disaster:

> WARMER OUTSIDE
>
> + STAGE LIGHTS
>
> + LAYERED COSTUME
>
> + HUNDREDS OF PEOPLE
>
> + MOVEMENT AND ADRENALINE
>
> = BUCKETLOAD OF SWEAT

I know, why in the world would I share an equation for sweat? Well, friend, this isn't because I wanted to show how much work acting was. It's because this equation led me to the moment my life changed.

Confused? Let me explain.

AUDREY MARIE

When I was spending six days a week sweating in the costume, I started to get odd bumps under both of my arms. Now, I had had that type of bump before, but never as many and never as big. I wasn't quite sure what they were, but they were painful.

What if it's cancer? I had a strong fear of cancer.

"They are cysts, honey. Don't mess with them, and they will go away," my mom explained.

That worked for quite a long time. I began to simply ignore them and pretend as if they weren't there. I assumed they would go away (just like every other time), plus my mind was busy with the play and school. I chalked it up in my mind that they were just weird armpit pimples.

Armpit pimples....

Does that even exist?

They never popped, and they didn't really look like pimples, but what else could they be? It's not like I've ever heard of cysts before my mom told me. As I continued the final weekend of my show, I realized that one particular bump wasn't going away. Not only this, but it was becoming painful even to set my arm down or shower. You will never guess what I did and what this led to.

The very last show was an incredible experience. But there was one thing that was distracting me from all the excitement. Pain. After the show and the celebration, I went into my mom's bathroom to see where the pain was coming from. It was a stabbing, burning pain on my right armpit. I lifted my arm and saw the bump had a tear-looking mark on it. So, as most would, I squeezed it. I mean, all that could've done is get rid of all the puss (I know. TMI). I also really thought it would help the pain. This was the moment when that bump opened. I wish I knew that the lump would refuse to close.

I quickly walked downstairs to show my mom. My mom appeared concerned when she looked at the lump. You know when moms try to avoid showing you their fear, but you can clearly tell? Yep, that was the look my mom made. The very next day, we went to the pediatrician's office. The minute I lifted my arm, the doctor said exactly what my mom had said a few days prior.

"Oh, no, that's not a pimple. It's the remnants of a cyst".

I was absolutely disgusted and embarrassed. I almost felt dirty or as if I didn't take care of myself. But that's when he said the two words: Hidradenitis Suppurativa. This was the first time (and definitely not the last) I would hear of the condition. He proceeded to explain that I needed surgery on it pretty quickly since it was becoming infected often. The cyst turned into an abscess-like wound, and it wasn't going to close on its own.

AUDREY MARIE

The doctor then explained that he would send me to the best surgeon at the major hospital in Richmond, Virginia. So, I went home with nothing but devastation, fear, and bad news.

PART TWO
life-lasting moments

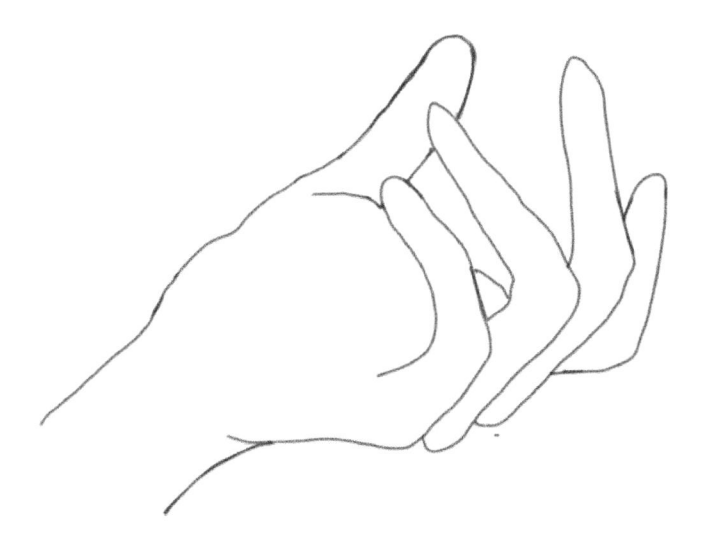

Chapter 6

And the Process Begins...

The night before my pre-surgery appointment was restless. I knew I wasn't going to a hospital to be evaluated, but that didn't help much because I didn't know what my future held. Being referred to a major hospital typically means you have something serious going on. And although I'd had broken bones, fingers slammed in doors, and concussions, none had required a well-known hospital franchise or a specialist.

I stayed up that night and had a conversation with God. "If you make this go away without surgery, I will never do anything wrong again. I will pray multiple times a day, never cuss, and always say the Rosary." I was attempting to bargain with God.

I tried my hardest to promise whatever I could to take the stress away. But that's the thing about religion and faith—it's not about making deals or promises. It doesn't only appear when you are desperate or need something. But 16-year-old me didn't know that. It would take many more lessons to learn that life-changing fact.

• • • • ● • ● • • •

All appointments can cause stress. It doesn't matter what they are for. For some, the dentist can even cause sleepless nights. Fear and distress are all relative. But the stress of this appointment was unmatched in my life.

"Maybe it won't require surgery," my mom said on the way to the appointment. "It could just be an in-office procedure."

Every part of me didn't believe her. I had a feeling there wouldn't be a quick fix for this painful lump in my armpit, which had become red, swollen, and constantly oozed yellow liquid. It hurt to sweat, put my arm down, get dressed, shower—or do anything and everything. The armpit is such an awkward area to have even a cut on, let alone a large bump with an opening. Still, at this point in the process, I was willing to deal with the ailment instead of facing surgery.

Maybe it'll go away, I thought. Or, *Maybe it's just something I will have to deal with*. But I knew deep within that I couldn't live with this pain and discomfort. No one should have to live with pain lurking like a shadow—right?

So I walked into the small office, looked around, and proceeded to wait for my name to be called. As I slowly sat down, I could hear the creak of the chair beneath me. I put both arms on the cold, metal armrests and uncomfortably hung on. Almost like I was on a cliff trying not to fall. My breath was shaky, and I couldn't sit still. There was no music playing, just the sound of the receptionist talking with my mom as the smell of sterilizer permeated the air. I was about ready to run when my mom finally came and sat beside me with a clipboard.

"How tall are you?"

It sounded as if she was underwater.

"Uhh, 5 feet, 2."

"How much do you weigh?"

The questions my mom asked felt like they went on forever. Right as I was becoming distracted by the interview, I heard my name.

"Audrey Marie."

With a huff, I stood up as if irritated instead of stressed.

After the routine checkup by the nurse, we were sent to an examination room. I climbed up on the classic table—with a tissue-paper-like cover—and waited. I knew that the surgeon would come in and give me the news. Maybe my mom was right. Maybe my gaping wound would require just a quick in-office procedure to close it up. My brain was trying any and every way to bring myself to peace. It was already trying to protect my psyche from what was to come.

But there was no way to prepare for the future I was about to have. The future, which would be set in motion the very moment the surgeon walked in.

He was tall with a charismatic stature. He wasn't dressed how I assumed a surgeon should be dressed—I guess they don't all look like mad scientists walking around holding a scalpel. He sat down on the circle chair with wheels and asked what was going on.

I told him the entire story. It was short and to the point.

With one look at my armpit and a few pushes to examine the lovely liquid, he quickly determined I needed surgery to get it to close.

"But this can be a quick procedure here, right? Could you even do it today and get it over with?" my mom asked with a trembling voice.

The surgeon looked at us both and laughed. "Absolutely not. This needs to be treated at the hospital in Richmond. She also needs to be completely under anesthesia."

My heart sank. I didn't know what to say. I never had surgery before.

He then grabbed his clipboard and, on the back of some useless paper, drew out what he would do. He explained exactly how he would cut into me, what he would try to take out, and then the testing that would be done to determine it wasn't cancer.

...wasn't cancer....

I never thought of that as a possibility. *There's no way it could be something that serious, is there?*

The ride home was rough. I remember just crying out of fear. My mom was unsure how to help.

I can't go. I can't do this.

Everything about the idea of surgery scared me. Even the thought of IV needles frightened me, let alone ones that insert a form of plastic in your arm. As I write this, I understand that my experience was pretty normal. Many people are scared the first time they go under anesthesia. A lot of people are afraid of needles or even pain. But you, my new companion, will soon see my experience was the furthest from normal.

Chapter 7

Take My Problem and Double It

The two weeks before the surgery flew by. There were moments of stress and fear, but I frequently forgot that the surgery was coming up. That was until the pain from the haunting open lump under my right arm reminded me.

"When you get through this, we will buy you a fish tank," my grandparents promised.

Something about fish and aquariums has always been so calming to me. Staring at an aquarium brings sudden peace. It is important to know what brings a level of peace into your life. Without it, life can make even the calmest lose their sanity.

Although I was terrified, I was hopeful that it would all be over once I finished the surgery. I was ready for my life to get back to normal. It didn't matter how much people promised me; the greatest present would be having my skin closed. I would finally be able to shower, sweat, and do everything without pain. What a thought!

We must see the positives, my friend. In the meantime, at least I still had one arm without pain, right?

At last, it was just 24 hours until the surgery would begin. Terrifying thoughts went through my head: *How bad does an IV hurt? What does it feel like to be "put under"? Will I dream the whole time?* Questions most people who go into surgery have. So far, my journey had been entirely normal. That was until I woke up a day before the surgery with a fear of something hovering over me. A feeling I had become well acquainted with.

I walked into the bathroom to do the standard check of my armpit when I felt something weird under my *other* armpit. With my stomach on the floor, I slowly lifted my arm. *This can't happen. I can't deal with this right now.*

I rushed to my mom to show her the giant boulder lodged in my left armpit. It was a painful lump that couldn't be denied.

Immediately, my mom called the surgeon. "What can we do? Is there a medicine for this?" I heard the shakiness of her voice. "She is in pain, and I don't know what this is."

The surgeon answered with a sentence that may have set my life on its course. "I will take that one out tomorrow as well. It won't be a big problem."

I couldn't believe it. There's no way that, within 10 minutes, I went from having one arm cut open to both. How can we blame him? Surgeons are paid to perform surgery. To them, it isn't a 'big deal.'

• • • • ● • ● • • •

As I write this today, I understand that signs should never be disregarded or ignored. Still, I can't blame myself or my mom for missing this sign. How were we supposed to know that determining whether to perform surgery should never be done over the phone? Maybe the sign was that the surgeon would be neglectful. Potentially, we would have asked for a second opinion. But let me ask you this: What is the point of regret? It won't serve me now.

Chapter 8

No Explanations

I woke up incredibly early on the morning of surgery—which was good since the surgery was scheduled for 9:30 am. I put on a bra and t-shirt, grabbed my headphones, and headed to the car. No matter what, I would blare Miley Cyrus' *Bangerz* album and pretend like nothing was happening. My entire family followed and piled into the car. We had to drive an hour south to get to the large hospital in Richmond.

It was the longest hour of my life, and I could feel the stress coming from my mom and siblings. This time, I couldn't be strong for them. We arrived and all crowded into the elevator, pressing the floor number for surgery. I can still remember the sound of the elevator as it passed each floor.

After checking in, I was taken into a private room. I remember saying my age, "I'm 16," thinking I shouldn't even be at a children's hospital, let alone be scared because I was 'practically an adult.'

The nurse just laughed and said, "Well, 16-year-olds still need their mom." I rolled my eyes and went to sit on the bed.

"Oh, here, before you sit down, change into this." The nurse handed me a robe, grey socks with smiley faces on them, and a bonnet-looking hat. I went right into the bathroom and got changed.

As I came out, my mom was talking with the nurse. They were laughing and going on about how stressful this can be. My mom was asking one billion questions that were related to my safety coming out of surgery. I just had one single question: *Will anything hurt?* I jumped into the standard hospital bed and nervously shifted my weight around.

"Would you like a numbing shot before we place the IV?" the nurse asked as she sat in a chair next to me.

Numbing shot?

"Where is the IV going to go?" I'm sure I sounded anxious.

Once the nurse explained why it needed to be placed in my hand, I quickly agreed to the numbing shot.

Remember when I said I was terrified of needles? Well, let's just say the numbing shot stung worse than any bee sting ever could. This was the first moment I had to be truly strong—on a different level, of course. In the blink of an eye, the IV was in, my "bonnet" was on, and the surgeon was coming in to see me. The next thing I knew, I was preparing to have sedation and miss the next hour or so—or so I thought.

My hospital bed was rolled down a cold and empty hallway. There were so many people dressed in scrubs and blue hats. I looked up and read the clock—9:42 am. *I'm still awake. Am I supposed to be asleep?*

Suddenly, we went through tall doors into the operating room. I don't just mean the room you are sedated in; I mean the most sterile room you can possibly imagine. There was a nurse standing right over me. "Do you see what's all over the ceiling, Audrey?"

I looked up and saw stickers all over the ceiling—princesses, superheroes, and Disney classic cartoons. They were not as distracting as I would have liked. "Kids love to look up and see all the different cartoons. They always tell me what their favorite one is."

You bring kids into this room AWAKE?

"Okay, Audrey, we are going to start the sedation. Start counting back from 10."

10...9...8...7... I started to feel incredibly tired. But I was suddenly being lifted off the bed. Four different people on all corners of the sheet under me lifted me calmly and placed me down. The surface beneath me was hard and very uncomfortable. I realized fast that I was on the operating table. That's when the panic set in.

I'm supposed to be asleep. There's no way they would put me on the table awake. They need to know I'm awake.

They began strapping me down with three thick, black straps—one around my ankles, one around my waist, and one around my arms.

Oh...my...gosh....

My world then went black.

Chapter 9

Not That Bad

"Hey Audrey, how are you doing, honey?" I opened my eyes to a nurse typing on a computer and my mom staring straight at me. I had never felt stranger. I remember realizing that I felt no pain.

That wasn't that bad.

My family came in and gave me different presents: stuffed animals, fidget toys, you name it. I also got apple juice. Aside from what I remember, I've been told I was incredibly goofy. I was telling my typical jokes and chatting with the nurses. Honestly, I was pretty happy. That was until I was told that I needed to get dressed.

"Audrey, we can help you if you need it. You will be wobbly; why don't we go into the bathroom."

Pshhh I can do it.

I thought I knew better. This was the first time I felt something unnatural under both my arms. When I went to lift my arms to put my shirt on, I could feel thick bandages lining the crease of my armpit.

That feels weird.

I now know what I felt. It wasn't that any pain was there. I simply felt uncomfortable. That was until I got in the car with my mom's assistance. Once I was helped into the chair in the back of the minivan, my mom reached around me to put my seatbelt on. This was the first sign of PTSD.

• • • ● • ● • • •

My dear friend, I believe it is essential never to doubt your body or impulse reactions. My reaction to the seatbelt in the car only hours after being strapped to the operating table showed that I was having a trauma response. How was I supposed to know? How are we ever to know we are being warned by our body? My body was about to betray me in the worst of ways. I quickly learned not to trust it. I still don't. I don't know if I ever will again.

• • • ● • ● • • •

As my mom went to put my seatbelt on, I panicked. The sudden fear rushed through my mind and body.

No.

No.

This can't happen again.

What can't happen again?

I didn't remember quite yet what had happened to me right before being put under. All I knew was that being strapped down in any way—even with a simple seatbelt—couldn't happen. After crying and fighting my mom, the seatbelt finally clicked.

"You're okay, Audrey." I could hear my mom's exhaustion. "Let's go home."

We were on the way home when I got my first taste of the pain I would soon become familiar with. Pain with a sensation I can't express. A sensation that something was inside my body. You see, when you hit a pothole in the road, your body tenses. It's an immediate reaction. What happens if your muscles tense, but there is something blocking them from tensing completely?

• • • • • • • • • •

AUDREY MARIE

I know, I know, I don't want to get ahead of myself here. I can say I wish I would have cherished the next 24 hours. But how was I supposed to know what was waiting for me the next day? I think that is a lesson we always need to learn. We don't know what tomorrow will look like. God does that for a reason. Let me ask you this: If you already know the major plot points of a book, do you still read it with the same passion and excitement? That's kind of like life. Tomorrow may hold a major plot point in your life, so you might as well live passionately today.

Chapter 10

Calm Before the Storm

Several events surrounding the surgery will forever affect me.

The surgeon wanted to say it would be simple—a fast procedure. "I do these all the time," he said. "It'll be standard and a pretty quick fix."

Since this came from a doctor, that was the mindset I went in with. I left that hospital in Richmond, Virginia, with a positive outlook on my future. I remember the nurses and surgeon giving my mom the aftercare instructions—but I didn't really pay much attention.

Who cares? I won't feel it.

Little did I know the very next day would change the wiring of my brain. It would be the defining moment that tested just how strong I really was.

AUDREY MARIE

How strong should a 16-year-old be?

• • • • ● • ● • • •

I woke up the next day with pain in both my arms. But as long as I didn't lift them at all, my armpits didn't hurt. So, I stayed on the blow-up mattress my mom set up the night before and watched cartoons. (Yes, *Scooby-Doo* is my comfort show.) I didn't go a second without oxycodone in my system. I couldn't function without it since the surgery had been less than 24 hours prior. Honestly, with the medication, I wasn't in *that* bad of shape.

I remember being incredibly goofy from all the meds. Still, I had a weird feeling in the back of my mind. Every time I shifted, sneezed, coughed, or moved at all, I was reminded of my condition and that I still required care for my wounds. *If I don't think about it, I won't have to worry*, I reasoned.

The day passed by in the blink of an eye. I was still sitting on the mattress in the same location when my mom walked into the living room. "Let's go upstairs and get it over with," she said.

I knew exactly what she was talking about. My stomach dropped.

"The doctor said we can do it easier if you are in the bath."

CHRONICALLY UNSTOPPABLE

Easier in the bath?

I took a big gulp and slowly walked up the stairs. My mom quickly gave me oxy again to help with the pain. I quickly asked, "What do you have to do?"

My mom looked at me with fear in her eyes—a level of fear so deep even she didn't realize she was showing it. "We just have to take out some of the bandages so we can clean the wounds."

My heart began to race. I started to sweat, and my knees buckled. No one wants to have their wounds touched the day after the surgery, and I knew this wasn't going to be any average aftercare.

Twenty minutes after taking the oxy, I walked up the stairs. I could see my mom in the bathroom. As I wobbled in, she started the bath.

"Why do I have to get in the bath instead of just standing here while you do it," I quickly asked.

My mom swallowed and said very calmly, "The surgeon said it will come out easier."

Come out?

I was already feeling the effects of the pain medicine, but it didn't prevent me from questioning what exactly that meant.

At that point, I started to put two and two together. Whatever this was going to be, it wouldn't be easy.

• • • ● ● • ● • • •

Even as I type this, I can feel my heart start to race. My mouth is getting dry, and I am beginning to shake. No one should have to go through something like this. Still, years later, I feel as if I am in that bathroom waiting for it to happen. But don't stress, friend, this is exposure—the exposure I need.

• • • ● ● • ● • • •

My mom recommended I take off my clothes, get in the bath, and put a towel over me. She waited outside, and I slowly shut the door. I looked in the mirror and breathed.

I can do this. It is super-fast, and I won't feel it. Just pretend like you aren't afraid.

I turned around and put one foot in the water. Everything in my being screamed, *No!* But I had no idea just how difficult my immediate future was going to be.

• • • ● ● • ● • • •

Sometimes, people don't remember when their fight or flight moment kicked in. I shut something off in that moment. Was it my emotions? Was it my present mind? Seven years later, I still don't know.

• • • • • • • • • •

My heart dropped as my mom walked in. My arms were practically glued to my side as I submerged myself in the bath. The idea of water on the wounds sounded worse than the pain I had already experienced. But please, dear friend, don't seek a comparison of pain as you read this. Pain is relative. That is something we, as humans, need to learn. Typically, we try to relate to things to understand them better. I had nothing I could relate the pain of this experience to. That's all you need to know.

My mom knelt on the floor next to me. "Okay, lift up your arms so water can get to your wounds, honey." (She always called me "honey" when she had something upsetting to say.) After a long argument and battle, I finally lifted my arms, dousing my wounds with water, and then quickly lowered them again.

Wow. I didn't feel that at all. My altered brain was thrilled and couldn't believe it. I very quickly began to gain hope.

Sadly, what I didn't realize was that water did not get into the wound. You see, it was plugged. Plugged like a cork in a bottle.

"Ready?"

I slowly raised my right arm.

• • • • ● • ● • • •

I believe some moments change the course of history. Maybe that date who stood you up actually set you on a trajectory to meet someone better who was waiting for you. Perhaps because nothing seemed to be in your corner, you stepped out and found a faith to believe in. Positive or negative, there are moments that change the course of your life. I'm only 23, and I can say I've had enough life-changing moments for a lifetime. Don't get me wrong, friend; I am not lecturing you on "everything happens for a reason." Upon reading advice like that, my younger self would have thrown this book right in the trash. No one wants to hear that they were diagnosed with a disease because it would "help them become a better person." If you ask me, that's all wrong.

Instead, think of it like this. Our life moments are a series of dominos. The 50th domino cannot fall if the first domino doesn't. Some may take longer to topple because they are farther down the line, while others might fall in the shape of a curve. The moment I am about to describe to you was a domino—a very large, heavy domino. I wouldn't be sitting here today writing to you if it didn't fall. Did it make multiple dominos fall at once? Without a doubt. But just like the rest of the sequence, one event led to the next, creating the path of my life.

Here is my trigger warning. I will be talking about intense post-surgery wound care. If you will be triggered by this, please do not read it. Skip to chapter 12.

Chapter 11

Brain-Changing Trauma

There I was—16 years old and in a bathtub, holding my arm up high. A moment I never thought would happen. My mom slowly reached toward my armpit. I assumed it was a small ball of cotton that she would need to remove.

I'm okay.

This'll just be a second.

I felt my mom start to pull. That is when the nightmare struck. I realized she kept pulling. Think of it as that trick where the magician pulls a ribbon out of his sleeve, only in horror movie fashion. I could feel every length rub against my wound. It felt like years until it finally all came out. I slowly turned my head and saw the longest piece of gauze I had ever seen in my life. It was covered in who knows what. All I could do was cry and scream at the horrific pain I felt in my armpit.

CHRONICALLY UNSTOPPABLE

Don't get me wrong; this is not to scare you. I am not attempting to have you cringe at my book and never read another thing I say. However, I want you to realize the impact this had on me—the impact it would have on anyone. After feeling the pain erupting in my first arm, I started to "check out," or, as my therapist would put it, "dissociate." My mom began to tear up as she attempted to convince me to lift my other arm.

"It'll be so fast. You can scream as loud as you want."

I will spare you the gory details of the screaming and pain. But I need you to know this forever changed me. But not just me. My mom and everyone in the house felt the effects of my pain that day. The fact that all my family heard this happen is worse than you would ever imagine. Remember when I said I was the protector and strong one of the family? Well, this illness finally forced me to show colors I never wanted my family to see. I think that is why this had to happen. The experience forced me to be protected by my family. Well, as protected as I could be with something not in their control.

• • • ● ● ● ● • • •

I thank God I made it through that. No one in their life should have to go through medical trauma like this without any professionals.

However, this is what I would like to point out. We are in a society that believes medical professionals know all. We are taught not to question and only follow blindly. From the moment I saw the operating room to my experience in the bathroom, I never once questioned the surgeon. He was (and still is) the chief head of surgery at a major hospital system in Virginia. Sure, I was 16. But please listen to me.

No matter your age or state of being, you are the expert in your life. You get to decide what procedures are done on you, and you get to ask all the questions. When we make the decision to follow blindly, we agree to sign over the control of our lives. I am still paying for these societal standards, and I don't want others to go through this. Empower yourself to speak up. Follow your gut. It could save your life.

• • • • • • • • • •

Once both pieces of gauze were out, I stood up and got out of the bath. My entire body was shaking, tears were rolling down my face, and I couldn't make use of my words. I slowly walked into my mom's bedroom and lay down on the bed. You see, it wasn't over. My mom had to put a light bandage over the wound. Nothing else. No ointment, no gauze, just a bandage over two holes in both armpits.

Let me pause here and ask you a question. Would this be proper practice to have someone perform wound care at the home with no medical supplies? I guess that is up to the interpretation.

I only saw the surgeon a couple of times after my operation. Once was within the week of the surgery to see how I was doing.

"You seem to be healing well," the surgeon said after a quick glance.

Physically or mentally?

"The immediate aftercare was pretty rough for her and me," my mom attempted to put into words what I simply could not.

The surgeon laughed. "Yeah, I guess it can be a hard one."

He guesses it could be a hard one?

I guess surgeons get to become desensitized to what we cannot. Oh, plus it didn't physically happen to him.

• • • • ● • ● • • •

That was the first time I experienced invalidation from medical professionals. No one realizes the damage this does to someone. I pray to God that you, my friend, haven't gone through this, but if you had, words can't express how sorry I am. Many people wondered if I felt anger in that moment. But that is the thing when you take away the voice of someone who never had one to begin with—they never want to speak up.

• • • • • • • • • • •

I must be weak. This is something that happens all the time. I'm a wimp.

I'm a wimp.

I am a wimp.

That was the day I decided to start silencing myself. I stopped complaining and talking about the situation as a whole. I told myself I was wrong to complain. That was, until I saw the opening in my right armpit had no sign of healing. Again and again, my mom emailed and called the surgeon.

"This is typical. Keep treating the wound. It will heal."

Unfortunately, there was no treatment to be done. It only consisted of changing the band-aids and wiping the wound with a tissue.

How long should someone wait? Are we to follow mindlessly indefinitely? Unfortunately for me, my time went well over a year. A year of treating a wound, going to high school (leaving class to go into the public bathroom and change my bandages), dressing in costumes for theater, exercising...all with an open wound in my armpit.

I wish I could've been there for you, Past-Audrey. I wish I could have told you to scream until someone opened their ears. Beg until someone offered help. But I can't go back in time. I won't. But I am here for whoever is reading this. Now is the time for you to take a stand for yourself. Then, in the future, you can go to your past self and give them a huge high-five.

Chapter 12

Here We Go Again (Just Successful)

After pressing the surgeon, he finally decided to send me to a colleague. This time was entirely different. I walked into the hospital pavilion in Richmond, Virginia, more anxious than I had ever been. I was now suffering from the trauma I had experienced a year prior, and I did not know what was wrong with me. Within ten minutes of seeing the new surgeon, she suggested another surgery. That was the only way we could clean the wound and then get it to close. She left, and the nurse took some pictures of the wound. To say I was scared is an understatement.

• • • ● • ● • • •

I was a senior in high school when I had my second surgery under my armpit. We had a lot of faith in my new surgeon.

She took time with me—explaining what would happen and expressing her concerns.

This is something I want to note to you: Never be confused at your medical appointments. Everything a doctor diagnoses you with or does to you should be explained to you.

I have a lot of regrets for not taking the time to get educated on my conditions. Now, to be kind to prior me, not a single service provider offered the education I now advocate for. I recognize this as one of the most significant issues with the medical system. Patients should be educated about any condition or disease they have. The best way to get through a diagnosis is to understand not only what, but also how. For example, how you got the condition. With CRPS, education is crucial.

So please, dear friend, ask as many questions as you have. Request further education—but *don't* Google it. Please.

· · · ● · ● · ● · · ·

Our trust was rightfully placed in the surgeon; my second operation was successful. There was no aftercare trauma that could have been prevented, and eventually, the wound closed. I did, however, go through several months of trauma-inducing wound care. For example, I went for a follow-up, and the surgeon realized that the wound wasn't really closing. She picked up something that looked like a black match and explained that she would be cauterizing it.

"It will burn. You can cry, and mom, hold her hand."

God help me.

As I felt the stick roll over my armpit wound, I could feel an unimaginable pain. I couldn't help but cry. It felt as if my armpit was getting burned with fire (ha, ironic, considering I later got CRPS). This time, however, I had a tool I had developed—I checked out while it was happening. Is that a healthy tool? I can tell you that I didn't care at the time. Maybe I still don't.

I held my arm up so the wound could dry as my mom drove us home. The pain continued as the air dried the black substance now in my armpit.

Wound care like this repeatedly happened over the span of several months. Meanwhile, I was also enduring other health concerns. Past-Audrey was certainly struggling, going through something I swore I would never deal with again. However, this also wasn't the only thing I was dealing with.

I ask you this: How many struggles can a person take at once? Please know I am not trying to scare you or make you squirm in whatever chair or exercise machine you are reading this on. I am simply trying to get you into the headspace I was in. That is the only way we can learn. We have to know where we came from in order to know where we are going.

It wasn't long after the second surgery that I started to feel odd. There was more pain than I had ever felt, and it was all in my shoulders. *Both shoulders.*

"You've been through an intense surgery. Of course, you're still in pain," my mom said. "You've been so strong this whole time. Give yourself a break."

Although the pain was different, I didn't think to question my mom another time. That was until I was sitting in first block math class.

Chapter 13

Fire Ignited

"Ladies and gentlemen, I will pass out homework for you to work on," the teacher expressed as she grabbed the stack of papers off her desk. She had given me that nice teacher smile since she knew it was my first day back after the surgery.

I slowly reached behind me and grabbed a pencil out of my purse. It was a plus that, due to weight restrictions, I could only bring my cute purse to school instead of a heavy backpack. My friends commented about wanting to have what I have so they could bring a purse to school. I laughed and just shook my head. I liked that kind of dark humor.

"Do you know how to do number 1?"

I guess my friend assumed I would know even though I had been out of school for a couple of weeks. I grabbed my pencil and slowly put it to the paper. I immediately stopped.

CHRONICALLY UNSTOPPABLE

What in the world?

My shaking hand and arm made it hard for me to draw a single line. Not only this, but the pain was immeasurable.

Do you know what it's like to feel pain radiating from your armpit? Not just any pain, pain that is deep to the bone—like a fiery needle being plunged into a frail bone that is ready to crack. This was the first time I had felt pain like that. I knew it was different from the surgery pain—I just didn't know why it was different.

My brain and the pain made it feel like I couldn't write. No matter how hard I tried, my brain had already decided that writing was causing that level of pain. So, I began writing with both hands. At least I could hold the pencil steady, even if it hurt. You see, I started shaking. Shaking, which couldn't be controlled and made me feel so weak.

I looked over to see if my friend noticed. I know she tried to pretend like she saw nothing, but I know without a doubt that she saw the moment it happened.

The moment I felt the first touch of hell.

Over the next week, more symptoms came about quickly and without any warning. They engulfed me, plunging me into a pit of fear and pain. Within a few weeks, my own personal hell was created. My body and mind could not keep up with how fast I was declining.

The first consistent symptom (aside from the pain) was my extreme weakness. It felt like my arms and hands couldn't hold up a single feather. The simple task of getting up and walking to the bathroom made me feel like I was running a marathon without any training.

I also began experiencing tremors—shaking. First, the tremors would occur only when I was doing small tasks. Then, they happened more often. Finally, I was shaking for most of the day. Early on, this was just frustrating—I'd faced a lot of worse events in my life. But, within less than a month, I struggled with everything throughout my day, including getting ready, writing, eating, and showering.

My most critical and terrifying symptom continued to be the pain.

I know. Pain is subjective. We all go through pain. But again, I encourage you to take your comparisons out of it. This type of pain couldn't be handled by even the strongest person. It was a combination of burning, stabbing, and cramping—a deep pain that caused so much trauma it made me have trouble mentally functioning. It even raises my heart rate writing this now.

The pain started around my armpits and then spread down my arms to the tips of my fingers. It felt like my body was giving up on me. Shutting down. As if it were dying. No one should have to feel this way, especially a 17-year-old kid.

That is the thing about this pain—it doesn't kill you; it simply tortures you. The idea that I could have a disease forever did not make sense to me. Once the pain started, my doctors tested me for every disease in the book. Anything that could *possibly* cause the symptoms I was experiencing. If they found another disease, I reasoned that at least it could be treated in some way, right?

Out of all the tests I had, two of them brought me absolute hell. The first one is well known—I had to get an MRI on my whole upper torso. The medical professionals wanted to make sure that no lumps or tumors were obstructing my nerves.

I was in the tiny tube for an hour and a half. Then, on top of that, it took me about 30 minutes after to push through the psychological torture that came with it. My head was covered by a hard cage, and my arms were strapped down—the same way they were strapped down at the beginning of my first surgery. Basically, I was trapped and put in a kid-size tube for far too long. As a result, I still experience claustrophobia to this very day.

Test number two required so much strength and courage. Remember when I said I was scared of needles? I can say I got over that quickly with this test. I don't know if you've ever heard of it, but an EMG is a beast of a test. It typically comes in 2 stages:

- Stage 1: Shocking you with electrodes to see if your nerves react.

- Stage 2: Shoving a long needle into your muscle and then making your muscle move by flexing or moving a certain part of your arm.

I know—not a very scientific explanation. But this is exactly what the test was. It was painful. The needles were so long. And remember, simple flu shots were scary to me.

This type of test was my worst nightmare. It required so much strength and distraction. But I used the "checking out" I learned from my PTSD experience. I lay there and felt as if I checked out of my body. This was my way of coping with events that caused fear. My pain tolerance was becoming high ever since I developed those horrible symptoms. So, I was able to get through it. Not only that, but I still had an opening under my right arm that I was working with the medical team to close ever so slowly.

After the test was administered, I sat down on a chair next to my mom, waiting for the doctor to come in. To say I was nervous would be an understatement. I knew she would say I had something wrong, but what was it? My family and doctors assumed that nerves had been hit as my mom had removed the gauze a year prior. Despite their assumptions, there was still stress in the back of my mind.

What if I have nothing?

What if I'm making it up?

As I heard the click of the door, the doctor walked in. She sat close in front of me, holding a single manilla folder. She opened it to show the numbers that came from the test. She began to explain how normal my numbers were. As she spoke, my eyes filled with tears. This was my last chance at getting a diagnosis and help.

It was at this exact moment that the doctor leaned forward and said, "I understand this pain is bothering you. I would suggest you seek a therapist to help you through it."

I'm done.

I want to preface my reaction by saying I had a misinformed mindset about therapy. I thought that it was solely for people struggling with mental illnesses. So, I questioned, if I had physical symptoms, why would a doctor recommend therapy?

Oh. I reasoned. *I'm crazy.*

AUDREY MARIE

• • • ● ● ● ● • • •

The car ride home was difficult for me and my mom. I took all my fear and pain out on her. Was this fair? Absolutely not, my friend. But there was no stopping me. I was stuck in a car dealing with emotions and exhaustion for over an hour, and she was in my line of fire.

"I'm done, Mom."

"I'm crazy."

"This is all in my head, and I give up."

"I don't want any more appointments."

"No more time wasted."

"I'll get over this."

"I'm fighting this alone."

I'm fighting alone.

I could see the fear in my mother's eyes—not only the fear that her child was sick and in pain but the fear that I had given up. Not only did I feel helpless, but she also felt helpless.

I can't imagine being a mother and seeing your child go through something like this. We as a society often focus on the individual enduring the illness but often do not address the needs of the family. My mom had to watch as I slowly gave up. She tried everything she could, and yet nothing was enough. I am forever grateful that she never gave up on me. I don't know if I would be writing this today if she had.

Chapter 14

Complex Regional Pain Syndrome

We went back to my original neurologist when all the tests came back. I already knew she would say they all showed that I was perfectly fine. But this would be the first time I ever heard my diagnosis. My neurologist leaned forward and said the words: "Complex Regional Pain Syndrome."

To me, those words immediately sounded like a cop-out diagnosis. With the pain I was feeling, I assumed I would've heard that I had something horrible. Now don't get this twisted—it's not that I wanted to have a horrible disease, but being diagnosed with one would validate all I had been going through. Validation that what I was feeling was real and urgent.

Once I heard the diagnosis, my head immediately dropped. As someone who had usually been strong for everyone else, I couldn't hold the tears back. The doctor did not take the time to explain the condition to me. Instead, she said physical therapy and psychotherapy would help. Other than that and medication, I would need nothing else. Again, none of this matched the death I was feeling all over my upper body.

Therapy.

A shrink?

I had absolutely no words.

How would you respond if someone told you therapy would fix horrific pain? I'm sure you'd have a few words for them. That was the first amount of doubt I experienced in my journey. I rode home with my mom, screaming at her the whole way out of frustration and fear.

"I'm crazy. I'm beyond crazy. None of this is real. Just forget it all. I will deal with this on my own, and it will go away. Just get me a shrink."

Desperation.

Fear.

That is what CRPS does to its victims. Doctors can play a big role in how a diagnosis is received. That specific doctor did me a disservice. She instilled in my brain the thought that I could control the pain. In other words, I could simply will away my pain by dealing with the anxiety and fear. Having the knowledge I do now, I know there were a million other ways the medical team could have handled the situation. I wish I had known it then. Maybe it would have saved me some of the emotional pain I was about to face.

• • • ● ● • ● • • •

Within the week, I began going to physical therapy. My evaluation was somewhat depressing. My strength was so low that some of the test tools couldn't even get a read. I was constantly tremoring from my shoulders down to my hands. The physical therapist (PT) questioned whether or not I had nerve damage despite all the tests clearly showing I did not.

"This could take years. The amount of damage to your system is concerning."

The PT struggled to understand my condition and ended up getting the head physical therapist. Even he was stumped. I remember so vividly the moment he told me, "This is going to take years potentially to get you better." Was that a good decision for him to tell me that? Who knows.

Immediately, I disagreed in my head.

No possible way.

CHRONICALLY UNSTOPPABLE

• • • ● • ● • • •

This is the first important thing I've learned throughout my long battle: No matter how rough things may get, you must believe in the deepest part of your soul that you will win. Does that mean I didn't have doubts? Absolutely not! There were times when I believed that my life would always be miserably painful. But there was something that always told me not to give in. I thank God every day that I didn't. Sure, people are going to give up on you in life. Sadly, even many whom you believed to be the closest to you. But you can keep going without people. You can't keep going if you lose yourself. Remember that.

• • • ● • ● • • •

Next, I was introduced to a physical therapist assigned to help me. I would end up having physical therapists who would do me more harm than good, but this physical therapist was one of the only medical professionals I learned to trust during this time in my life.

Mary was a young PT who supported me no matter what. During my appointments, she would talk about life. Never once did I feel like she thought I was crazy. Nor did I have to defend the pain I felt. It is crucial to understand, my friend, that when you have an invisible condition, it is typical to feel weird at appointments. I had lost my trust and faith in medical professionals when I experienced my trauma after the surgeries. You will later find out how poor physical therapists can adversely affect someone like me. But for now, let's be positive.

Mary worked with me every week for many months. It was crazy difficult. I was so weak that I couldn't even lift my arms above my head. My wound was still healing, and I still had plenty of restrictions.

Although the sessions felt like they were as long as the previews at movie theaters, there were some moments of fun.

"Okay, the next exercise is cat/cow."

Cat...cow...?

I was not going to do that.

Mary laughed as I explained how ridiculous it sounded. We had so many moments of laughter. Looking back, I see how much her cheerful demeanor and intentional conversation distracted my pain and anxiety.

Not long after I started with Mary, we determined I needed occupational therapy. Within two months of feeling that first touch of pain, my hands had become incredibly weak and began to curl. Slowly, I began using them in a claw-like fashion. That certainly needed to be addressed, but I had prior beliefs about occupational therapy: I assumed it was only for people with severe disabilities. I mean, that wasn't me. Right?

Surprisingly, occupational therapy with Sarah wasn't that bad. Although the actual activities were difficult and often frustrating, I looked forward to spending time with Sarah. We had plenty to talk about, and she had the same sense of humor as me. Not only this, but I could see the pride in her eyes when I did a challenging activity. With her, I never felt weird or like a puzzle. This was a huge deal.

You see, my dearest friend, when you have conditions not often seen by medical professionals, they tend to look at you like a child looks at a monkey in a zoo. I know you may have felt that way at some point in your life. But let me ask you this: what would happen if you felt that way every day for five years? Eventually, you would start thinking that you were so different that you deserved to be scrutinized.

Sarah and Mary were the only medical professionals who looked at me like I was an everyday person. I just had some struggles. Don't we all?

Chapter 15

My Pain is Related to What?

I fought for my life senior year of high school, and let's just say I was losing rapidly. I was attending physical and occupational therapy twice a week, every week. Not only that, but I had also gone on homebound for several weeks. For those of you that don't know, being on homebound is when a child does school from home due to a specific circumstance. It took forever to convince my neurologist that I needed a break from attending school in person. But the fact was that after arriving at school, I would throw up even before attending first block. And then I would sleep through the rest of the day.

My mom got the message one night after I came home from school. My pain was through the roof, I still had an open wound, and I told my mom between sobs, "I can't keep doing this, Mom. It hurts."

"Well, what do you need?" my mom said with a voice that sounded desperate and on the edge of breaking.

CHRONICALLY UNSTOPPABLE

What do I need? Did I even know at the time?

"JUST HELP ME."

The amount of desperation I felt was at a level I had never experienced before. It was as if every trauma, every second of pain, bubbled up into this moment. I didn't know how or when, but I knew I needed help. I don't know where I would be if my mom hadn't taken me seriously. She could have chalked it up to me being a dramatic teenager. Based on what most medical professionals were saying, I was okay. Nothing was life-threatening. Not everyone has a parent who listens to them above everyone else. Thank God my mom was one who did.

• • • ● ● • ● ● • •

I know what you are thinking, my friend. Not another break in the book where I explain what Present-Audrey thinks of Past-Audrey, but I feel that this is important.

I can't imagine the position our loved ones must be in. Sometimes, they must decide whether to follow the doctors and everything they say or, instead, to ignore that sought-after medical advice and keep pushing to find other help. In life, we learn lessons. My mom would say she learned many throughout my journey.

We need to, for lack of a better term, cut our loved ones some slack. It can be difficult for them to know when to yield to a doctor, especially when they aren't the ones experiencing the physical pain. For this reason, it is so crucial to have open communication. Even if you want to give up and stop asking for help, give an extra push. That one added request may make a life-changing difference.

• • • ● • ● • • •

While I was on homebound, I had a teacher who truly cared. She was there to support me but also gave me the grace I needed. Don't worry, I earned every grade I got, but I got as much time as I needed to complete assignments. During this time, I struggled to complete even a single worksheet in one sitting. One primary reason is that I would fall asleep at random times. I know you may be confused. I sure was. Let me explain.

At this point in my life, my body was struggling. I was still heading to the hospital constantly to attempt to get the surgical wound to close, experiencing a level of pain that was unspeakable, and rapidly losing my mobility. I put it this way to show you that my mind, body, and soul were exhausted. The more stressed I would get and the more pain I would feel, the bigger the threat was to my nervous system. This is when my body started a forced shutdown. Weird, right?

This type of shutdown looked as if I was simply falling asleep. One minute I could be crying or tremoring, and the next, I would be completely asleep. This could happen in a store, in the car, in class, at my house, with friends—you name it. It was happening to me many times a day. I was completely and utterly terrified. I couldn't control it. And I still experience it today. My friends and I call it a simple reset. We must learn to joke about things. That's the only way I could get through it.

I was close to graduating when my neurologist pressed that I get a therapist. My mom had shared that I was going to school every day wearing pajamas and not doing my hair or makeup, which was incredibly out of character for me. Not only that, but I would also spend the whole car ride (since I didn't have the ability to drive myself) either screaming and crying at my mom or not speaking at all. It made sense that therapy would help with what I was going through.

However, my past self was furious that the neurologist kept pushing. Any time therapy was brought up in previous appointments, I'd refuse.

I don't need to see a therapist; I need medical help.

My past self didn't understand the trauma I'd had and was going through. Looking back, I recognize that anyone who has gone through even a few of my experiences would benefit from professional therapy. Finally, when I realized I needed to apply to college, I decided to listen to my neurologist. I was getting desperate, and it felt like time was running out. I needed to get 'fixed' so I could go away to college. That was my main goal at the time. I knew (or thought) nothing would stop that from happening.

I pulled up to the therapy office in an old brick building. I walked into the hallway, with its dimmed lighting and smell of essential oils. While some people might have viewed this scene as calming, it put me on the defensive. I had sat down for barely a second before the therapist walked out.

"Hello Audrey, why don't you follow me back," she said with the softest tone in the world.

Good Lord.

We walked into the office with a single chair and a sofa. Naturally, she told me to sit on the sofa and fill out a few forms for a questionnaire. This was the first time I needed to fill out paperwork without my mom present. The problem wasn't that I was nervous to fill it out; the problem was that I couldn't.

My ability to write was out the window, and my stomach sank through the shag-carpeted rug.

"I…uh…I struggle to write…uh…my condition…" You could hear the embarrassment in my voice.

"Oh, really? Hm. Interesting. Do your best to fill it out," the therapist said without looking up from her laptop resting on her portable desk.

Do my best?

Although this was the first time I had to reveal this particular struggle, it wouldn't come close to being the last. Until I learned to write again, I got weird looks from people. It didn't make sense to them that I would look so typical and then "claim" I struggled to write. I want to emphasize that we all have struggles, and the fact is, we owe no one an explanation. However, I also understand that although writing that in a book is easy, it is more difficult to live it out. I still wrestle with that.

That first hour of therapy went by painfully slowly, but there is one thing I would like to point out. During the initial evaluation, I was asked about my family structure. Naturally, I said I didn't have a dad around. That was when I got the response that would change everything. I didn't trust a single therapist after this very statement. That was, until I met the one that helped save my life.

"Have you ever considered, Audrey, that the pain you feel is related to the heartbreak and pain around your father leaving? Potentially, that could be why you were recommended to see a therapist."

• • • • ● • ● • • •

People don't realize that singular statements can make or break someone. Every word you say has the potential to remain on someone's mind for five minutes or five years. This statement was said to me when I was only 17. I am now 23. You do the math.

• • • • ● • ● • • •

You won't be surprised to learn I never returned to that therapist. I felt shame, embarrassment, and heartache—so many feelings, my friend. I could cry just thinking about Past-Audrey. I think that the therapist's statement was truly the catalyst for Past-Audrey's downward spiral. Although I can't go back and reassure her, I would like to reassure you. No matter what you are going through, you should never feel as if you need to defend your pain. Remember that you are your biggest advocate, but I am happy to be your number two advocate.

Chapter 16

Knock Back—Let Fly

By the time spring rolled around, I was spending most of my time in my bed. That was where I ate dinner, worked on homework, messed around on my phone—you name it. I wanted to move as little as possible because moving always made my pain worse. I wanted to exit my body—to take off my fiery skin and put on a new one. I felt stuck in a body that was burning itself alive, and I couldn't even stand long enough for a shower. I also began to realize that if I wanted to seek higher education, I would have to apply for and get accepted into the college that was only 10 minutes from my house. This was because I believed I could not live in a dorm. I could barely even function in my house with my mom helping me. And all the accommodations Sarah and I decided on were not my idea of a 'normal' college kid.

On top of it all, I soon learned that Mary was moving on to her next stage of life. Although I was happy for her and her growing family, I couldn't help but be disappointed. I didn't feel like I was at a point of not needing physical therapy, but I wasn't sure if I wanted to start over with a new therapist. Don't worry; you'll soon see why. My outlook on life spiraled as I felt like I had no purpose. I had nothing to motivate me or give me something to look forward to. That was until one particular day when I was riding in the car with my mom back from one of my many Richmond hospital appointments.

"I just have nothing to look forward to, Mom. Nothing to inspire me." My tone was incredibly calm.

"Well, YOU inspire ME."

What a mom-thing to say.

"Why don't you volunteer for the hospital, Audrey? Or even donate?"

Every time we would go to the hospital, I would notice the youngest kids. Often, they were there to get chemo or have a checkup for some disease. They were all so strong. You could tell in each and every one of them that they had a special gift. They had seen the most challenging parts of life at such a young age.

Seeing this got me thinking. I began researching what I could do to help these patients. I asked myself that if I couldn't find a purpose or something to look forward to from the comfort of my own bed, how must those kids feel? After many conversations with my family, my organization "Knock Back—Let Fly" was born.

I hosted an event at the local library where all my friends, family, and community members could build individual gift boxes filled with stuffed animals, puzzles, coloring books, crayons, and crafts. Then, we delivered that first round of boxes to the very hospital where I had experienced trauma a year before. It was powerful, exciting, and emotional.

"Why are you naming it 'Knock Back—Let Fly'?" Sarah asked me during an OT appointment.

"Because no matter what knocks you back, you need to let it be the catalyst to push you forward."

With an arrow tattoo pointing forward on my wrist and a passion for helping people in my heart, I continued fundraising for my organization. Sure, the pain and trauma pushed me back, but it also flung me further ahead than I could ever imagine.

• • • ● • ● • • •

I tell you about my organization so you understand this: Past-Audrey felt she needed a purpose to motivate her back to health. Sometimes, motivation is not a magic fix. However, motivation in some form is what often drives an individual to overcome a seemingly insurmountable obstacle. Not everyone needs to start an organization to find a purpose, but it is necessary to find a motivation that will help you hang on for dear life.

Despite all I endured, I graduated from high school with the certainty that I was going to college. However, senior year was different than I had imagined: I lost most friends, didn't participate in the senior play, couldn't go to the senior dinner dance, and endured so many more disappointments.

But there were some positives, too: I had started my own organization at only 17, gone to Disney World for the first time, met Sarah and Mary, and survived a fight most people weren't even aware I was fighting. I must say—I'm so proud of you, Past-Audrey. You did so much with such little life that seemed to be left in you.

Chapter 17

To Keep or Not to Keep Faith

The summer before my first year of college was extremely depressing. I had lost everything—my strength, my positivity, my hope—everything. Not only that, but Sarah ended up moving away and leaving the therapy office I went to. One of the only medical professionals I'd trusted was leaving in the blink of an eye.

"She can't leave before I am better," I told my mom with tears running down my face.

"She has her own family. You want her to do what she needs to do. Right?"

I was terrified that I would have to start with a new occupational therapist. I had been through many traumas and worked with medical professionals who disregarded my emotions. The stress was unmatched. Even today, I can say that the stress was rightfully placed. I would soon learn what it means to have damaging occupational therapists. Sarah not only had a passion for her job, but she also had a passion for helping me get my life back. Sadly, I wouldn't understand this aspect of her care for another few years.

I focused on the thought that I got into college, asking myself, so what? I thoughtlessly went through the motions to take the next step in my life. All I could think of was my favorite quote of the time: "Hope breeds eternal misery."

I know…it doesn't even seem real. I would joke all the time when I said it, but I knew for a fact that I actually believed it.

"If I'm not hopeful, I won't be disappointed," I told my mom. "It saves me even more sadness."

This was the moment I noticed I started losing to the disease.

As I said, CRPS doesn't kill you. Instead, it burns everything inside you and leaves just an empty box in the shape of a body. I don't even know how I can explain the world I was living in. All I know is that I was giving up.

Because I was unable to embark on the adventure of leaving home to attend college, It felt like there wasn't anything to look forward to. And there was no end to the pain in sight. This was a level of helplessness that had exceeded anything I had faced in my life—a helplessness that threatened to rip my faith away in a heartbeat. CRPS was consuming my faith and trust in God as fast as a fire can engulf a home.

• • • ● • ● • • •

Before I begin to discuss my faith journey in detail, I want to preface it with this: our faith experience is often like riding a roller-coaster. And as you will soon see, I was about to plummet into the depths as I began experiencing distrust and dislike for God. I can't tell you how dark of a time that was. As you read the details, you will soon understand why.

• • • ● • ● • • •

From the moment I was diagnosed, I began to question why this had happened to me. Once I realized blaming the surgeon was fruitless, I began to look inward. The first time I questioned God was when I was sitting in a pew in church.

"No matter what, God will always be there for you," I heard during a sermon.

Will He?

I experienced sudden anger. It caused me to put my face in my hands. I couldn't listen any longer. I couldn't listen to promises of love. Promises of care. If God loved me as much as they said, why would He allow me to get a terrible disease? The way I saw it, I had only two options when it came to moving forward with my faith:

1. Lose my belief in God altogether. Assume He has never been there.

2. Believe He must be punishing me, leading me to no longer have love for Him.

Not believing in God was never an option. It never made sense to me that nothing comes after we are gone. So that meant that God had to have been punishing me.

I am sure you are wondering what I thought God could be punishing me for. I had determined that it was because I couldn't protect my mother from my father. Even as I type this now, it does not make sense to me that I could be blamed for something someone else did. But that's the thing about CRPS. It quietly eats people from the inside out. It's the worst and best abuser ever to exist. The control and power it had over me was stronger than any human power.

After this thought took hold of me, I realized I was furious with God. I didn't want to go to church or pray at any time of the day—even with my family before dinner. I just couldn't do it.

I wouldn't show respect to a figure that I felt wasn't showing respect to me.

This is the thing with faith. It's easy to feel thankful to a higher power when things are going well. However, can faith be found when things are more difficult?

I look back and realize God was there with me the whole time. And He has grown me and my faith. In fact, I like who I am more now than I did before I contracted my disease. Because now I have the capability to understand people despite what they have gone through. I use this talent of empathy in both my job and everyday life.

But I'm not going to lie; the hell I endured is worth no amount of growth. Sometimes, we just have to make the best of what we are dealt. God challenged me, and I didn't have a choice but to accept.

Chapter 18

Stagnant Suffering

The next three years would become a fight of a lifetime. While writing this book, I spoke with my pain therapist.

"What came from those few years?"

Is she thinking negative or positive things?

"Do you want to know the good things that came of it?" I quickly asked.

"Whatever you think."

I don't know if I could put those three years into words.

So, I want to tell you a few stories that taught me lessons throughout those years. It took me until much later to realize these lessons fully, but I am grateful for each one. As I have said repetitively, mindset is everything. Once I was able to take a step back and reflect on each situation, I realized there was so much I could learn from it. I am hoping that you, my friend, will be able to learn from my life events, too. Maybe you won't have to live through similar events if you are able to read them here.

So, good or bad, here is a fast-forward of those next three years.

• • • • ● • ● • • •

Ages 19-21 are crucial for becoming an adult. During this time, you can learn essential social skills from every situation—from experimenting with parties to dating. But what happens when you spend that period of time fighting for your life? Do you just feel like you fall behind, or do you *actually* fall behind? That is the question I am still trying to understand the answer to.

• • • • ● • ● • • •

My original plan was to attend school to study theater. I loved theater and was confident I was good at it. So, it wasn't surprising that 'entry-level theater' was my very first class on my very first day.

That day, I met the one trustworthy friend I would have for the next four years. Noah was unjudgmental and never asked me questions. Despite my hands shaking or my necessity to record lectures, Noah saw me as a normal girl.

Asking people to help me write my name on a paper, which I had to do often, doesn't seem like a big deal. But words cannot express the looks I got when I asked. My request didn't make sense to them. I looked completely able, and yet I wasn't. College quickly taught me to keep my head down and avoid asking for help.

If you can relate to this, I'm so sorry. We should limit our judgments on people. How would those college students feel now if they knew their single reaction stuck with me for years?

Most of us have an idea of what our future will look like. It is no surprise to most that our plans don't work out too often, but this wasn't what I struggled with. There is so much more that goes into the emotional pain I feel for Past-Audrey. I was repeatedly invalidated by most people and organizations in my life.

You see, in the span of two years, I had gone through four occupational therapists at the same facility. Some of them were kind; others were not. Often, I was instructed to do a single repetitive activity for the entire hour. Sometimes, I was used as a test dummy for students who were there to learn, as the facility was part of a major teaching hospital. Every single occupational therapist made me feel strange. I felt as if I were a lab rat and they were simply testing ideas to use for other people. This brings me to my next point.

Some medical professionals struggle with arrogance. They refuse to admit they may not know the answer to something.

It was clear that all four of the occupational therapists who treated me did not have a clue about CRPS. Instead of letting me know that, likely afraid they would be doing me a disservice, they kept the façade up. I even had an occupational therapist get her school textbook and open it to the page that explained CRPS.

"Go ahead and read it so you get the idea," she said, barely looking up from her laptop.

There's no way this is how I should be getting help.

I was confident I had a somewhat good relationship with the physical therapist at the time. That was until I took a week off to go on a vacation with my family. You and I have become good friends since you made it this far in the book, so I will share this with you. But first, let me explain my insecurities at the time.

• • • • • • • • • •

When people have a widely misunderstood chronic condition, they often struggle to find medical help. This means that the help they find may be their only grip of control.

Please understand this: when someone is in this position, being forced to miss an appointment can cause a catastrophic setback. Please know if you feel this way, it is typical. It is understandable to have the sole focus of wanting help, of wanting the pain to stop. I would have done anything and everything to get it to stop.

• • • ● • ● • • •

I took a week to go on vacation with my family—a normal occurrence for most people. But it meant stepping out of physical therapy for a week, and I was not ready to take a "break" from my progress. So, on the way to the beach, I wrote my physical therapist an email outlining my plans for the physical activity I would be doing.

Part of the email stated, "...every day we are going to the beach...I will spend at least a half-hour swimming in the pool! I thought you'd be impressed with that one!"

My motive was simple. I was a young kid who wanted encouragement and to make someone proud. I'm sure you are wondering, 'So Audrey, what's the point?'

Well, you see, I never heard back from the PT that whole trip. I ended up assuming she was busy and just couldn't answer.

I didn't hear from her until I was in the middle of my next occupational therapy appointment.

"Hey Audrey, I got your email," the PT said with a serious face.

"Oh yeah, I assumed I got the wrong email address," I pretended, knowing she just didn't answer.

"I received it; however, I want to keep this relationship professional. I'm happy you went on vacation, but it was unnecessary to tell me."

I know you may be thinking that was a little (or incredibly) harsh. But with tears in my eyes and stress in my body, I thought of one single statement.

I'm crazy and obsessive.

When you've had so many judgments placed on you in life, you begin to internalize almost everything. I had gotten to the point where I convinced myself that nothing was medically wrong with me; I was just obsessing over the idea of going to physical therapy. I know. I even debated leaving that in here because it just doesn't sound right. But trust me when I say some people will get it, and to those people, you are not obsessing over medical treatment. You are fighting for a better future for yourself.

Chapter 19

Just Let Me Drive

It wasn't long after I got diagnosed that I started a bucket list. This list gave me a drive and hope that I was very much lacking. It was filled with things most people are used to doing in their everyday life.

Write my name.

Drive a car.

Go on a date.

It changes your perspective when you dream about things you once took for granted. I wonder if the bucket list was good for me. Sure, it made me dream and helped me find a hint of hope—but it also confirmed in my head that I wasn't successful when I couldn't do the things on the list.

CHRONICALLY UNSTOPPABLE

There are activities I still haven't done on my list to this day. Let me tell you a story about how I completed one of the items on my list: getting my driver's license.

• • • • ● • ● • • •

I had already learned how to drive with a permit before I was diagnosed; however, I got CRPS prior to getting my license. I tried so hard to push myself and take the driving test, but my body wouldn't allow it. It's a hard lesson to learn when you realize that there is nothing you can do; your body is shutting down. I have to say this had severe effects on my mental health. How would you cope with losing the independence you were so close to gaining? I know. No right answer.

I spent almost five years with the inability to drive. My older sister, Emily, drove me as often as possible to high school and every day to college. Although I spent most days crying or yelling at her, I will be forever grateful for what she did for me. She didn't have to do that despite what I was going through, and she tried every day to make me smile. Those days of smiling may have saved my life.

We began searching for alternatives to typical driving techniques by the time I was 20. That was when we found a state disability service that would assist with any training and adjustments that needed to be made to the car itself.

• • • ● • ● • • •

Let me make a note to you. I struggled with the idea of needing to do anything different to drive. I didn't want to be labeled as disabled or even need accommodations on my wheel. It made the condition too real for me. Especially when I was doing everything in my life to avoid the truth: that my body was under attack and I might need a little extra help.

• • • ● • ● • • •

I was lucky enough to find an adult resource institution in Virginia that would not judge me. They didn't question my abilities and why I was struggling to use my hands. Within a few short months, I was getting my license at the DMV thanks to my new steering wheel equipment. This opened up my world of confidence and independence. It gave me the exact pick-me-up I needed to keep going. I wonder where Past-Audrey would have been if she didn't gain an ounce of independence. Maybe she would have given up.

CHRONICALLY UNSTOPPABLE

I want to point out that I make videos spreading awareness about how I drive on TikTok. The number of hateful comments I receive is shocking.

"Just grab the wheel."

"Girl is faking for views."

"Good luck getting past a cop using those."

I wish I could take each comment and explain how they are wrong. Maybe educate them so they don't say hurtful things to a future young Audrey. But what I have learned is there is no use. People will make judgments no matter what you show. I apparently didn't appear to be suffering enough. It shows that we may not be enough for some people's views. All that should show you is who is safe.

Find your safe people in life. People who don't question whether you are sick enough or healthy enough. Instead, you are simply enough.

Chapter 20

Rilee

When I was only a couple of weeks into my first semester of college, I came across an individual who had a service dog for chronic pain. The dog knew when her pain was increasing and was able to keep crowds away, protecting the affected limb. As always, I will ensure you are caught up by explaining further.

You see, with CRPS, your skin becomes sensitive to the touch. As I write this, the thought of someone rubbing my arms makes me sick to my stomach, as the amount of pain I experience through touch is excruciating. Don't get me wrong; this aspect of the disease could be different for everyone—some people may not experience this symptom while others may experience it differently, for example, saying that hard touch is significantly worse than soft. But seeing the service dog gave me an idea of how I might be able to protect myself from pain. And since pain was a constant part of my life, I began researching.

My options for getting a service dog were limited. As you'd expect, there aren't a ton of dogs being trained to help people with chronic pain, and the very few that are cost tens of thousands of dollars and have a waiting list longer than the lines on Black Friday. So, my only other option was to adopt and then train my own service dog. How can someone with chronic pain who struggles to care for themselves adopt, raise, and train her own service dog?

Since you and I are friends now, I know you understand that I often don't choose the easy way out. To me, easy is boring. So, naturally, I decided to adopt a puppy and train her to be my own personal service dog. The first challenge I had was to get my neurologist on board.

"I wanted to bring up something that I think could help me." I was clearly nervous even to ask.

"I'm always happy to discuss options to help you!" the neurologist surprised me with her excitement over my autonomy.

"I recently saw someone with a service dog. I want one, and I need your permission."

After a long conversation, my neurologist agreed with one condition—that I get the dog and train her myself. I later realized that was because she knew the dog would get me moving and help me focus on something other than the pain. Within 30 minutes, my mom and I decided to get me a puppy. That's when I met the dog that would save my life.

The puppy I got was the last golden retriever of the litter. She was obviously the runt, but she was the sweetest dog I had ever met. There was an immediate connection. You see, when I was on the way to the breeder, there were three dogs left to choose from. But we ended up getting lost, and by the time we got there, only one dog was left. It was clear God meant for us to end up together. With tears running down my face, I took my first picture with Rilee. The name means "a strong and courageous women"—everything she would represent to me. I now knew I was no longer alone in my fight against the pain. Rilee would be with me no matter where I was.

Rilee was the most brilliant dog. She ended up going to college classes with me. It wasn't that she necessarily did physical things for me; instead, she distracted me from the pain. It took just a short period of time for her to start recognizing when I was struggling more. She would immediately sit right beside me so I could cry in her fur. When I was up at 2 am crying enough tears to fill a pool because of the pain, she would just sit and be there. Be there for me. Sadly, Rilee's fate was determined by her first vet checkup after I adopted her.

The appointment was going well. I was told how smart Rilee was and how much she was already watching my movements.

It was all smiles and laughs until the vet put her stethoscope on Rilee's chest.

"It appears there is a heart murmur. It sounds strong. Probably a grade 3. This dog will not have a long and happy life. If I were you, I would give her back to the breeder, who will most likely put her down."

This can't be happening.

My mom realized the situation and quickly asked if the vet was sure. Without blinking an eye, the vet said she was certain.

• • • ● • ● • • •

Life can be full of disappointments; however, it can also be full of beautiful moments.

When someone has a chronic illness, they can become more upset by negative things. This is due to the fact that it can feel like problem after problem is coming your way. As you'd expect, I struggled with this new news. But no matter what, I knew one thing: Rilee was sent to save me. Despite my disgruntlement with God, I knew she was an angel. And if she would never give up on me, why should I give up on her? So, Rilee and I made a pact. We wouldn't give up on each other. It didn't matter how scary or hard things got; we would never give up.

AUDREY MARIE

• • • • ● • ● • • •

Still, to this day, I know Rilee is one of the main reasons why I am as alive and successful as I am in life. She was the one who forced me up out of bed when the pain was chaining me down. She watched me with every ounce of her being and was ready and willing to do whatever needed to be done, even if it risked her severe heart. She was the fiery light in a world of darkness.

Sadly, Rilee passed away at just five years old. She passed while I was writing this book. Losing her was worse than any pain or sadness I have ever felt. I didn't know how I would go on without her. But I can tell you as I type this with tears falling on my keyboard, I know what I fight for today. I know WHO I fight for. I spend every day making sure I am making Rilee proud. It brings me so much joy to know she is in heaven, running with a healthy heart. I am sure it brings her joy to see how I am continuing to get up. Even though I can't physically see her, I know she is right here, and boy is she proud.

RIP Rilee Oyiyia

Chapter 21

Show Me I Can Do It

It is not unusual to try to find people like you. We, as humans, like to put everything in a box or category. It becomes even more prominent when you feel abnormal or odd compared to your peers. After being diagnosed, I quickly became desperate to find people like me. I wanted to see someone living happily with or after CRPS. So, one night when I couldn't sleep and the pain was taking over, I began googling:

> "My life with CRPS"
> "Living with CRPS"
> "Beating CRPS"

The list went on and on. No matter what, I could find very few social media posts. And all of them were about how the individual was bedbound, doing infusions daily, or had amputated their affected limb. I couldn't watch these videos. They were, in their nature, negative. It made me sick watching that, wondering if that was my future. Instead, I wanted someone to look up to, but I was struggling to find someone. That was until I saw a particular YouTube video.

As I was crying, I looked at the right sidebar and saw the video titled "What It's Like To Be In a Coma" by a girl named Claire Wineland. As you'd expect, it grabbed my attention, and since I was giving up finding someone with CRPS, I clicked the video.

Something happened when I clicked the video. Yes, of course, it was incredibly interesting. However, it was something about the girl talking. She seemed to be right around my age (maybe a couple of years older), and she had a disease called Cystic Fibrosis.

Within the blink of an eye, hours had passed, and I was still watching every video and Ted Talk she ever did. I was absolutely fascinated by how she spoke. Claire was in and out of the hospital and slowly losing her lungs, yet she was so happy. It made no sense to me. Why does she seem like she is doing amazing things despite having a horrible disease that is slowly killing her?

• • • • ● • ● • • •

People get placed in our lives for a reason. They are there to teach a lesson about life and make us grow. I was desperate for someone to show me hope. I thought someone could speak to me only if they were dealing with my exact situation. But Claire, who was dealing with something completely different, ended up giving me hope by sharing her story, and she never knew it. What an amazing impact we as humans can have on each other.

• • • • • • • • • •

Several quotes made my eyes fill with tears as I watched Claire's videos. One was from a talk she gave. She said, "We cannot keep teaching people who are sick that they need to be healthy before they can live their lives." At the time, that concept made no sense to me. We can't live while we are sick. I had spent the last few months waiting for my pain to go away, waiting for the time when I could start living again. Yet, Claire had been sick her entire life and still lived an incredible life.

Finally, I had found my person to look up to. The person who understood that suffering *and* living could coexist.

As I went to put my phone on the nightstand, I quickly exited out of the internet tab. As I did that, I saw a news article posted only a couple of hours earlier. Claire Wineland had passed away that same day from a complication with a lung transplant. All within the period of a couple of hours in the middle of the night, I felt excitement and then grief.

Claire was someone that I aspired to be. She was positive and had an amount of wisdom that isn't held by many. It is so important for us to have a couple of Claires in our lives. We need people who can show us that life is possible. Despite what your circumstance is, you can find the beauty in life. People don't need to have the same exact life as you in order for you to connect with them. Often, our connection has to do with the general spirit and feeling of the person.

I am grateful that Claire showed me how to make something beautiful out of everything life throws at me. However, I don't want to give you the wrong impression. I didn't magically decide to start living alongside my pain. But I did start to question if hope breeds eternal misery. I began to wonder if it instead breeds eternal beauty.

Chapter 22

Rally Around Me

Being diagnosed with CRPS not only disrupted my life but also disrupted my family's life. Thanks to my mom, our family was always incredibly close. Now, the person who was the protector of all needed protection. Not only this, but my family did not fully understand my condition. If I didn't understand it, how could I ever expect them to? Although they weren't experiencing the physical pain I was, they were going through the emotional pain of seeing me wither away. I knew this, and I have to say, my friend, it hurt me to know I was causing them stress and despair.

We all hold specific roles in our lives. However, events may require us to take on other roles and others to take on the roles we held previously. My mom was up night after night researching my disease and looking for treatment centers. I always refused anything that required me to be inpatient. "I'm not bad enough for that, Mom." My words came across like I was angry, but in reality, I was absolutely terrified. To protect myself, I would self-sabotage to avoid any more disappointment. I assumed that because a doctor hadn't recommended inpatient care for me, then clearly, I didn't need it.

• • • ● • ● • • •

I have to take a moment and tell you—If you feel like there is a treatment that could potentially help you, ask for it. The person who knows you and your body best is yourself. I have a condition that many doctors do not even know exists. That means those who do know may not know about all the treatments available. If I know you as well as you know me, then it may make you feel weird or obsessive to ask for a specific treatment. Don't let your brain, pain, nervous system, or anything else trick you. There is nothing odd about advocating. After my experiences, I will be saying that forever.

• • • ● • ● • • •

Our entire family structure shifted. No matter what was happening in their lives, my family surrounded me with support. It didn't matter if I was yelling from the pain, throwing up, falling asleep in a store, or experiencing any other symptom;

my family was there. Most of the time, I could see the pain in their eyes. But as I want to continue sharing transparently, I will tell you I did not always handle this support very well. More often than I should have, I yelled with frustration at my mom. I encourage you to please remember that type of treatment isn't fair to those who support us. My mom was often faced with my worst attitude; my irritability from the pain and hopelessness needed a target, and she was it.

I've learned, my friend, that no matter what is going on in my life, I have no right to treat someone poorly, even though I couldn't yell at the disease itself and I am imperfect. I learned that when I snapped at people, it was on me to apologize. I learned to take time to explain what I was going through, doing my best to help those who were supporting me understand where I was coming from. One thing for certain, despite my missteps and the misdirected anger, I'm grateful that no matter what I did, my mom stuck by me.

As I grew up and grew through my illness, I became incredibly close with my younger sister, Olivia. She was about 15 when we became best friends. The most important thing Olivia did for me? Not once did I see her look at me with sadness or as if I was a science experiment. On days I needed more help, she didn't blink an eye. No matter how many times I would snap at her, she explained that it wasn't fair for me to do that. If she wouldn't get a pass, then neither would I. I felt normal around her. I mean, don't get me wrong, we spent most of our time together laughing. Remember when I said we all have gifts? This is one of Olivia's gifts. I believe God gave her this gift in part so she could be there for me.

My other siblings—Emily, Robert, and Gia—were there for me as well.

Emily drove me to and from college daily, even though I refused to talk to her. She also watched Rilee when I needed her to and would buy me drinks and other things to brighten my day.

Robert was always there for me at night—night was my least favorite time of day. My pain was horrible, I often got sick, experiencing intense swelling. I wanted to be alone and cry by myself, but Robert knew that wasn't the best for me. So, he would talk to me for hours about topics he knew I cared about.

Gia was ready to help me with anything and everything. No matter how angry I was, I could see the readiness in Gia's eyes to help me no matter what.

Do I tell you all this to brag about my family? Absolutely not. As much as I love them, this is not what this book is about. I tell you this so you can understand an important concept: There are various types of support we can be given. Some are more obvious than others, but *all* are so important. Support does not only mean finding a cure or stopping the pain. Sometimes, unfortunately, that's not an option. The piece that all types of support have in common. They never leave.

PART THREE
finding hope

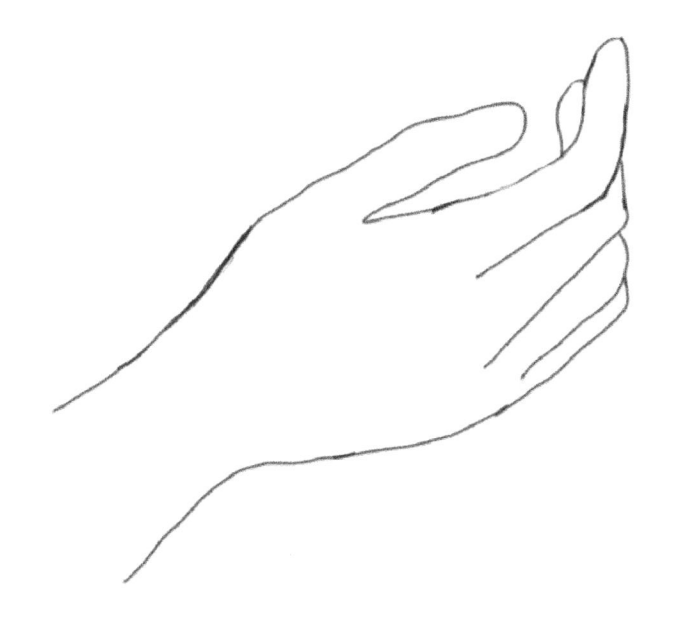

Author's Note:

Prior to reading this section, I want you to understand that everyone's healing journey looks different. Of course, I believe I found the best hospital in the world. But that doesn't mean you can't find one, too. It is all about mindset and finding people who get you. You'll soon understand.

Chapter 23

Waking Nightmare

My eyes opened as I looked around at my surroundings. Although I could see, everything was pitch black. I felt as if I were in a deep, dark prison with no way out. I knew I needed help.

"Help! Anyone. Please!"

No response.

"I'm hurting! I feel sick. Help me!"

As I turned around, I saw my loved ones. My mom, sister, doctor. They all stared blank, devilish stares.

"Why won't you help me?" I yelled with tears flowing down my cheeks.

No one flinched. No one cared. No one would help.

AUDREY MARIE

I woke up covered in sweat and tears, my hands squeezing my arms. Completely alone. Just as the nightmare told me, no one could help the excruciating pain in my arms.

You're okay, Audrey. You're ok. Just a dream (more like a nightmare).

• • • ● • ● • • •

Most of my mornings began that same way. It set quite the tone for the rest of my day. My family finally got the hint that asking "How'd you sleep?" was more than just a conversation starter.

"I hate when you ask that," I explained to my mom one day. "Just assume the answer is bad."

You see, when a majority of your days start off after a painful, terrifying night, it is hard to have a positive outlook.

Pretty soon, your days begin to simply pass you by with little joy.

There I was. I blinked, and three years had sped past me.

Sure, I had a lot of things going for me. I started applying to the FBI, got my service dog, made a few friends, and would soon graduate from college. I'm sure you are thinking, *What better place could I be in?* On paper, my life sounded wonderful and perfectly on time with the average masses.

But if I told you my thoughts and how I actually felt, you'd send me to the ER.

It was at this point that I lost most of my hope. I had searched everywhere for people like me—people who had been in the depths of their pain and had come out on the other side without surgery and pain medication.

What am I going to do? Nothing. I can do nothing.

I started to accept the fact that there was no non-invasive answer to this pain. I would have to give in if I wanted to live a happy life. I would have to do more than just therapies and limited pain medication.

I started researching ways to stop the pain. I recognized there is an extensive list of options, all the way to amputation.

I can't amputate both my arms.

I assumed I would follow the advice of my doctors. That was until I walked in for a rehabilitation appointment.

As my mom and I sat waiting for the doctor to come in, we heard the clock.

Tick tock.

Tick tock.

We looked around and saw patients coming in and out of a single room holding prescriptions. They had smiles on their faces. I had never seen something like this before. There were no nurses, the walls were bland, and there was only one doctor in the entire building.

"Audrey, you can go on back to the room," the secretary at the front office announced.

What in the world?

We walked into the room and sat on the two chairs. Within 20 minutes, the doctor came in.

He had a short stature and was on the older side. I was unsure of his understanding of CRPS, but he assured us he had treated individuals with the disease.

"Yes, it is clear you have Complex Regional Pain Syndrome."

I didn't know we were questioning it.

"I would be concerned about the clawing of your hands. However, that must be due to pain. What I would recommend is Oxycodone."

CHRONICALLY UNSTOPPABLE

Just like that? You will give me Oxy?

After I had taken Oxy after my first surgery, I had sworn I would never take it again. In just a short time, I could feel my body becoming addicted. It was my escape. This was a dangerous game I had been playing at just 16.

After he stated his recommendation, the doctor grabbed a pen and an empty script and asked a question I will never forget.

"How many prescriptions would you like? And how many pills do you want per day?"

Is this doctor really asking me how much Oxy I want?

Should I say that I want it?

He will give me whatever I want...

I quickly responded with a simple no.

You see, my friend, Oxycodone could not be on my list of options. I knew I was getting close to giving up, but I could not get swallowed up in the pits of addiction. I wouldn't. We all have our lines. Oxy was mine.

AUDREY MARIE

I want to clarify something. I do not judge the use of opioid medication for pain. In many cases, it can help people more than anything else. However, there is a way a doctor should go about prescribing any medication. The way this medication was dangled in front of me was tempting. I could have chosen to treat my pain with opioids, but because of my past experience, I feared I would become addicted. And I wasn't willing to take that risk.

• • • ● • ● • • •

So, despite the doctor's recommendation, I refused to manage my painful journey with opioids. Still, it was tempting. Who wouldn't want to check out of reality if their reality is pure pain and suffering? The question then became, how do I numb the pain I was experiencing so I could start living again *without* becoming addicted? I found the answer to all my prayers with a single appointment. Or so I thought.

My mom and I walked into the hospital with tension in our bodies. The words labeled across the large building read "Johns Hopkins." This was the first time we had gone to any northern hospital, and it was only our second time in Baltimore, Maryland. We were hopeful, figuring we would be offered different treatment now that we were outside of Virginia.

CHRONICALLY UNSTOPPABLE

The doctor walked in with a smile on his face. He spoke very quickly, not giving much of an explanation about anything he said. He reminded me of a surgeon in that way. I'm sorry, my fault. Let me correct myself. He didn't remind me of *a* surgeon, but of *the* surgeon who had played a huge part in the catalyst of my life struggles.

Although this doctor didn't want to change my medication, he did tell me about another treatment. And this was an offer I struggled to refuse. You see, my friend, he told me about something called a Ketamine Infusion. He explained that the procedure would take only a few hours and that I could sign up immediately to be put on the ever-growing waitlist.*[1] Even as he explained it with limited thoroughness, I knew this was more invasive than I would've wanted. But I was tired. Tired of fighting for just the littlest bit of life.

I had heard of Ketamine in my lifetime. It was on an episode of "Criminal Minds." I remember hearing that it was some tranquilizer that also caused hallucinations. I know, I know. It doesn't sound like something that should be put in a human's body. But I was desperate. And when my doctor told me it works on the pain receptors in the brain and explained, "It could make you pain-free for months," I desperately agreed.

---

1. *Please keep this in mind. It will come up later in the book.

I do question the thought process that comes when people are this deep in pain and suffering. Should we be told to make decisions for and by ourselves when we are so desperate? Oftentimes, we don't ask questions because we can't think straight. Then, on top of that, many people don't have family who are supporting and sticking by them. We need advocates. People who we can bounce ideas off of and know our questions prior to the appointments.

• • • ● ● • ● ● • •

As I said, the waitlist was long, and my patience was wearing thin. I could not wait until the day when I would be infused with the anti-pain juice. Sure, there were things to consider. There are intense side effects, and it is a daylong procedure that could make me feel even worse. But hey! Who cares! If it comes with the possibility of feeling no pain and living my life, I'm good!

What would you agree to, to feel no more pain? How desperate would you be?

Weeks went by; my mom began to side against me doing the infusion. After a few Google searches, she realized just exactly how this treatment could affect me. But no matter what it would do to my future, I wasn't going to change my mind. I refused to do research into the infusion. I was terrified of what I would find. But in all reality, you see, it didn't matter what the infusion would do to my body; I felt it couldn't be worse than the ongoing pain I was enduring. Plus, the only way I would start living was by getting the pain to stop. Or so I thought.

A couple of months after the infusion was scheduled, I went to see my neurologist. When I asked his opinion, he responded very strongly against it. Since you are my friend, you know that my trust in doctors was lacking, but I was gaining confidence in this particular neurologist. His beliefs fit with mine regarding what I was and was not willing to try. Oh, and he also said he dislikes it when neurologists don't believe in CRPS, saying with passion in his voice, "As if CRPS is something to believe or not believe in. There is literal proof."

It's a shame that these were my standards for what I considered to be a "good" doctor, but that's where I was at.

We left his appointment with only more questions, although he did explain in depth what infusions can do to the body. Once I had the full view of the infusion, I couldn't avoid the truth any longer. It crossed lines I wasn't even aware I had.

So, when I got the preparation call, I quickly told them, with tears in my eyes, that I had decided against the infusion.

"I just can't do it," I said between breaths. "There isn't enough research on it."

Now, what was the next option? I had just forfeited my opportunity for that treatment and knew it would take months to get an appointment if I decided to get back on the list. Yet I knew I couldn't live the way I was for all my life. I refused to allow it.

This is something important to remember. Chronic pain can take everything—your thought process, body, hope, and even religion. But please know all of that can come back. You need to be able to visualize your future. Even if the light within is the size of a single ink dot, there is always the potential for it to grow. That's all I needed. To hang on to the speck I had left.

Chapter 24

We All Need Support

I remember lying in bed crying the night after I canceled my infusion appointment—the doctor's words ringing in my head.

"Without doing the infusion, I would recommend raising your medication dosage significantly."

Meds, meds, meds. That's all everyone wants to do.

It was beginning to feel like a band-aid on a wound. Underneath, the damage remained. It was just partially covered up. Every day, I felt as if I were hiding my pain and suffering, pretending I was doing well. But my life was passing me by. I was breathing. My heart was beating. But I wasn't truly living. My real thoughts? Well. They looked a bit like this:

I only have a year until I graduate college.

I can't work like this.

AUDREY MARIE

I barely eat.

I can't live alone.

I can't.

I can't.

I can't.

The monster of "can'ts" took over my life. I didn't care that I was going to get my degree or that I was still making money babysitting and tutoring. It was all a lie I was living. People with chronic pain or any type of invisible illness are the best actors.

What if I told you we don't have to fake our way through life? What if I told you there is always another way?

I heard of another way from a girl in a support group on Facebook.

It was a morning of typical scrolling. I was in bed and reading through Facebook. As I was about to get off my phone, I noticed a girl posted on the "Ferocious Fighters" support group about a clinic in Baltimore, Maryland. She wrote that "The Kennedy Krieger Institute understands us." I laughed as I read the full post.

Sure. Just like all the other hospitals, medications, and procedures.

She went on to explain that treatment was done naturally and without pumping anything into her system. The only catch? It was inpatient care, requiring a hospital stay.

Oh. Heck no. I was not interested in inpatient care. Still, something had to give.

Without my mom knowing, I sent a private message to the girl. I didn't want to get anyone in my family's hopes up. I knew she would tell my siblings and grandparents (the most important people in my life). I was tired of hearing how they were certain it would work out. I had heard it so many times before. I wonder if they knew I could see the stress and fear in their eyes. I knew they were beginning to wonder how my life would turn out. Should they continue to live without me? Were they ever fully living knowing their sister/daughter/granddaughter was suffering?

After speaking with the girl for a while, I decided KKI (Kennedy Krieger Institute) was worth a try. I went to my mom and told her about this "miracle hospital."

Without pausing for a single breath, my mom simply said, "Okay." She has always been amazing like that. She never gave up on me, even if I was giving up on myself.

My mom spent a month getting the paperwork together. It took so long even to get an initial evaluation with the institution. In the meantime, I was struggling. I couldn't catch a break with the pain and humiliation I was experiencing.

Stressed about school? Pain.

Overworking just to feel productive? Pain, tremors.

Up all night due to lack of sleep? Suffering.

It felt like a never-ending, unrelatable struggle. I tried my best to cling to hope and people who showed a form of overcoming. I was lucky enough that Bailey was one of those people.

You see, Bailey is one of those people who make you question whether limitations even exist. Without giving you her whole story, allow me to share a glimpse. Bailey has Cystic Fibrosis (yes, like Claire Wineland). She has had surgery after surgery while losing her hearing and other abilities. Yet, nothing stopped her.

How did I meet someone so incredible? Well, she guest-taught at my sister's dance studio. Not only this, but she has her own studio, called Company 360, which allows everyone to dance despite and *because* of any and all ailments that many would think make them "less than." After speaking with her, I learned that disabilities and illnesses should never hold me back. They should never hold any of us back. Most importantly, I realized I could have a family someday, even if my disease doesn't go away. That's a wild concept, I know.

Bailey also introduced me to Justin Baldoni, an actor, writer, and director. He streamed on Instagram live almost every night during COVID-19, and I have to say, I watched every single one. Sure, his starring role in "Jane the Virgin" made him well known, but that isn't where I knew him from. Justin knew Claire. That's when I was first stunned by his ability to talk to those with illnesses as if they were "normal" people. He is one of my main idols, and I could never dream of him knowing me. That was until I received a video when I decided not to get the infusion. When I decided to keep living with excruciating pain.

> Hey Audrey.
>
> How are you? I hope you are having a beautiful day. I wanted to make you a quick video and send you a little extra love today. Alright?
>
> Stay strong. You got this.

This may sound like a standard get-well, but Justin took time while sitting on a train/metro to send this video to Bailey to be given to me. What an honor it was to have someone who knows people like Claire and Bailey take the time to know me. Bailey and Justin are people who changed the trajectory of my life, and I don't believe they know it. I spoke with Justin more after that, getting different advice (including advice on writing this book). Bailey and I also keep in touch. I support her in every way I can.

During this time period, the sensational app TikTok began to become popular. Everyone was beginning to quarantine, and TikTok simply took off. It was at this point that I considered making videos myself. But what exactly would I make videos of? I'm someone who cares about meaning and having purpose. I'm sure at this point we know each other well enough for you to recognize that. So, another day of scrolling consisted of me landing on one particular individual, The Tia Bee Stokes.

Tia is a mom of five who was diagnosed with cancer right when COVID-19 began. She was quarantined in the hospital, fighting cancer alone, and decided to start making videos. Her videos began with a few dances. They then made their way to YouTube, where she did nightly lives. I connected with Tia just as I connected with Claire, Bailey, and Justin. What was the thing that caught my eye? Tia is religious. She remained religious even through her diagnosis, and she never appeared angry at God.

That's a thing?

My brain and eyes couldn't believe the sight. Someone who had been given a rough go at life still held on to faith. That is when it finally clicked. I am drawn to people who don't lose faith—no matter what that faith may be.

Claire never swayed in her gratefulness of life.

Justin had faith in people who were struggling.

Bailey never gave up on dance.

Tia? She never gave up on God.

I was someone who had lost faith in a lot of things, especially God. I refused to believe that someone so powerful would choose this for me. Not only this, but I had lost faith in medical professionals, friends, and some parts of my family. And I was losing faith in myself.

Let me ask you a few things, my dear friend. Did it matter that I didn't personally know the people I found to look up to? Was I drawn to those with a positive mindset because I was envious of them? Or did I want to be them? Or were they just people who allowed me to escape my reality?

I can say I think it was a little of all those things.

But through our journeys, it is vital to have people to look up to, whether we know them personally or not. Because when we recognize the positive in someone else, we can envision it in our own lives. And when we get stuck and can no longer see a positive future for ourselves, we need to find it in others. This can allow us to hang on with the last bit of strength we have left.

The point is not to compare your life with someone else's. That only results in damage to yourself and them. Instead, compare mindsets. How does yours differ from theirs? What can you incorporate?

I decided to begin making TikTok videos after I found Tia. I developed my content based on how these four people lived their lives. Eventually, I have to say, I began to believe the things I said. Here is what I pulled from each person:

- Claire gave off an energy that allowed her passion for the beauty in life to blossom.

- Justin provides compassion and gives meaning to every single word he says.

- Bailey puts on display that anyone can do anything.

- Tia never gave up on herself and her faith.

• • • ● ● • ● • • •

Please, no matter where you are in your journey, look for people you can look up to. We are not meant to go through difficulties alone in life. Maybe even consider borrowing a couple of these amazing people I found!

Chapter 25

Am I Behind?

I want to use this chapter in my book as a break to explain a very crucial concept. At this point, I began to compare where I was in life with where it seemed like everyone else was. I know, I've already made it clear that I had questioned my trajectory before with the whole 'not going away to college thing,' but now, this had become a major stumbling block for me. I'm sure you are slightly confused about why I need an entire 'break' chapter for this simple concept. After all, it isn't surprising that I would feel like I was falling behind and wasn't the same as everyone else. But trust me, this ran much much deeper. I hate to say it, but if I look closely enough, the repercussions are still within me.

During most of the first quarter of our lives, we are all told exactly where we are supposed to be and when we are supposed to be there. After we graduate, we are given a few optional paths, but they are still laid out for us. And what happens when we graduate from college or trade school or finally get that promotion we want? Typically, we, as humans, then rely on our peers to show us the next steps.

These milestones in life include the ever-growing question of when we should get married. Technically, there is no set time to get married, but if all your peers are getting married at 24, you will likely feel behind when you turn 25. A lot of people experience this level of insecurity. And what happens when you feel as if you are behind emotionally? I am not talking about having the right job or diploma; I'm referring to social and emotional maturity. It's a strange topic, I know. But I have to be honest here, friend, and tell you that I have felt socially and emotionally behind the curve in the deepest part of my core. And that hurts, almost more than the engulfed flames I feel in my arms.

Let's all remember that I got diagnosed with CRPS when I was 17. That meant my world veered. When everyone else was getting permits, I focused on getting pain relief. When everyone else was dreaming of their future, I was trying to get through the present. But more importantly in my developmental process, when everyone else was stepping into the world of dating, I was simply not.

For most, a lot of dating happens throughout the senior year of high school and college. And, once you are the age of the typical college student, you begin to do a lot of emotional/social maturing. This development includes things like going to parties, dating that well-known bad boy, drinking, testing clothing styles, and learning how to take care of yourself as you navigate cooking meals and doing laundry. Dealing with my illness 24/7 put me behind in all of those areas. You could say I missed out on the development of life because I was too busy trying to fight for my life.

I began to believe I wouldn't amount to much.

There is no one like me. I am so behind.

TikTok became a large part of my life. Whether healthy or unhealthy, I would spend hours scrolling and comparing myself to everyone my age. I was hoping and praying that one day I would find someone who was where I was in life. To be honest, I just wanted to feel "normal." I now look back and realize how I put myself on a close-to-impossible task. Social media is fake; people rarely show their true life (the ups and downs). That was until I scrolled onto a girl named Soph Mosca.

One day, as I was scrolling through TikTok, I stopped on one of her videos. I quickly realized she was my age, but she caught my attention because she had a following and yet still appeared like a "normal" person. I began watching her TikToks and found them entertaining, but I didn't think much of her page. After giving her a quick 'follow,' I continued scrolling.

The very next day, her newest 15-second video came up. I clicked the comments and saw someone mention her new YouTube video. Now, I have to be honest and say that I was curious. I quickly switched apps to YouTube and typed in her name. My phone filled with results from her channel. Out of curiosity, I clicked on a video entitled "...vlog...getting real...". This was the first time I found someone that appeared perfect who had the same feelings I did.

You see, Soph had a following and could make a mark on people. She had her own apartment and could afford her own things. Despite all of this, she still experienced feelings of being behind or lacking experiences. I was shocked. It was that day that I realized that we all can feel behind no matter how much success it appears we have. Yet again, I was validated by someone who had no clue who I was. I continue watching her videos to this day. She doesn't lie about life being perfect because it isn't. She shows the good and bad. That, I admire.

As I continued watching each video, I felt validated and seen. Seen by someone who didn't know I existed. Time went on and I began watching every video she posted, knowing I was safe. Safe to hear what she had to say without concern for my own mental health from the unavoidable comparisons. I have to be honest, I began watching her videos all day, every day, because, unlike my peers, she never acted as if she were perfect. What a weird concept for an influencer.

I watched as Soph grew in followers and success. I was always a more silent supporter with occasional tags on Instagram. That was until I saw Soph post that she was recently diagnosed with Diabetes. I could see the stress and fear in her eyes—a visual I was too familiar with.

In her post, she explained feeling like a burden to her then-girlfriend and her constant fear of the disease itself and that her life would change entirely. That's when I decided I would reach out.

Finding Soph on social media was not an accident. She helped me without ever knowing, and I would finally have the ability to make her feel seen and heard, whether she would see my message to her or not.

After her quick response to my message, I went back to silently cheering her on. She continues to share the ups and downs of her life. If only she knew that she validated me at a time when I couldn't validate myself.

You see, dear friend, I tell you this story to show that despite what you think about people, nobody's life is perfect. If we must compare ourselves, find someone who shows all parts of their life. Once you find them, hang onto them for dear life until you can hold yourself up. Who knows, maybe one day you will be able to pay it forward. I know that's my current mission.

Chapter 26

One Last Shot

My appointment at KKI came quicker than I had expected. As always, I began to stress the night before. It is safe to say that by this point, I had developed a fear of all doctor's appointments and hospitals. I've heard people laugh and joke about that fear, calling it "white coat syndrome," but it is very real and not something to take lightly. Along with plenty of other associations, my brain had decided doctors were not safe. Where do we go when we are sick if doctors are not safe?

My mom and I got in the car, ready to make a much longer voyage into new territory. On the way there, you could cut the tension with a knife. I could tell the incredible stress my mom was under. We both knew and felt the invisible timer ticking away to my graduation. My mom realized that her positive attitude and words would not stop the inevitable from happening. Her daughter was fading away. What mom could bear to see their child being ripped from their dreams? To be honest with you, I never would have wanted to be in my mom's or siblings' shoes.

Our drive up to Baltimore was 2 ½ hours. It was the middle of winter; I was between my junior fall and spring semester of college. As we pulled into the parking garage, I noticed something entirely different. Although I was stressed, I wasn't scared. I know, I know, what is the real difference?

AUDREY'S OWN DEFINITIONS
STRESSED: Being weary about the future, whether immediate or later.
SCARED: Wanting to avoid the future altogether due to concern of danger.

I stepped through the automatic doors and looked around. There were the standard positive quotes on the walls and typical security managing the front desk. After having my photo taken and filling out paperwork, my eye caught a fish tank on the other side of the room. Sighing a big breath, I walked over to stare at the fish, hoping I would suddenly gain the ability to switch places with them.

"Audrey Marie?"

I've heard this exact scenario way too many times.

One look at my mom, and we followed the women into the back.

"Wow, honey, your heart rate and blood pressure are incredibly high."

Duh, lady.

I have always tried to give everyone the benefit of the doubt. But I have to be clear that I was a pessimist by this point. It didn't matter how kind medical professionals were to me; I assumed they were judging me from the moment they read my name off the manila folder.

My mom and I were brought into the room, and the nurse explained what was going to happen.

"Audrey, this will be about a 3-hour appointment. We will have you see the lead pain doctor, physical therapist, and therapist."

Ready for a pop quiz, friend?

What part of that explanation would have turned me away?

If you said therapist, you were right!

The minute this was explained, everything in my body wanted to turn away. However, just like times in the past, I refused to give up. I had a feeling about this particular hospital, so I pushed on.

"That sounds great to us," my mom said awkwardly.

"Audrey, please tell me why you are here today."

Oh, for the love of God.

I told much of my story. Skipping the details of my surgery after-care, I quickly went through my history. To be completely honest with you, friend, I was sick of telling my story. I know, that sounds weird as I'm writing a book about it now. But I was sick of people questioning my life and my experience. It was getting too sad and too exhausting.

Once I finished telling my full story, we all heard a knock at the door.

"Audrey?"

I smiled, fighting frustration, "Hi."

"Hi, Audrey. I am the therapist you will be talking to today."

Done. I am done.

After my mom was told to walk out, I lied the entire conversation.

"How are you doing?"

"Fine."

"How is the pain recently?"

"Eh, fine."

I wanted the conversation to end as quickly as possible. Honestly, I wanted the day to end as quickly as possible. That was until Dr. Sam knocked on my door.

He was of average height, bright, and incredibly kind. The best thing? Not once did he look at me like a lab rat.

The examination and appointment with him went incredibly well. He watched me write, looked at how my hands worked, saw my posture, and discussed my pain. But not in the sense of "rate your pain on a scale from 1-10." Instead, he asked me how my pain was affecting my life. For the first time, a doctor looked into everything that was affected, not just what he saw in the moment. After finishing, he left to have a conversation with the team.

My heart rate picked up.

I was sick to my stomach.

I didn't know what I would be told, but I knew they were going to deny me.

This was when Dr. Sam offered something that both scared and excited me at the same time.

"Audrey, the team and I talked."

Here we go.

"We recognize how much of your life is affected by this. I want to start off by saying I am so sorry you are going through this. We can tell how much pain you are in, and we can tell how much you want to get it to stop."

With a sigh of relief, one word went through my head.

Finally.

"We all would like to offer you our inpatient program here in Baltimore. It is intensive but will address you and your life as we tackle this disease from all aspects. Let's get you feeling better and into the FBI." He had listened. He knew working for the FBI was my dream.

• • • • • • • • • •

AUDREY MARIE

That was a moment I will never forget. Pure validation. Not only that, but a recognition of how much I was struggling from people who had the tools and were determined to help me. If you are feeling lost and alone, friend, please know that there are people out there willing to fight with and for you.

• • • • ● • ● • • •

The rest of that day consisted of a tour of the inpatient program, going out to eat with my mom, and a lot of crying. I was so shocked and scared for my future, but not in the way I was used to. For the first time in four years, I was thinking about my future, including things like what job I would have and where I would live.

Chapter 27

Virtual Treatment

It took me less than a week to sign up for inpatient care at KKI. As scared as I was, I was prepared and ready to fight for my life in the most intense manner.

As I waited, COVID-19 hit its climactic point in the United States, and I was stuck in the house, struggling more than ever and sharing my journey occasionally on TikTok. My pain was out of control. I was shaking constantly and starting to feel the pain in my back for the first time ever. I was getting sick often and didn't know what to do. I now know that my symptoms dramatically increased because I wasn't moving as much, causing my CRPS to worsen.

Don't worry. I'll soon explain this medically, but for now, let's continue the story.

AUDREY MARIE

I was two days away from going to inpatient care when I got a call that would change the course of my life and future.

"Hello, is this Audrey?"

"It is."

"Audrey, I am sorry to tell you that insurance denied inpatient treatment. They stated that it was not medically necessary. Part of it is because you are still attending college."

Because I attend college, I am not as 'bad' as I need to be?

I immediately broke down. This was my chance at freedom. I remember feeling completely defeated. I couldn't handle the pain that now overwhelmed me. Only this pain was different. It was entirely emotional. I had suffered through intense physical pain but knew I couldn't go a day with this new mental anguish—knowing that help existed for me but was out of my reach. You see, although I had become accustomed to the pain and suffering, the deepest parts of my soul still wanted my pain-free life back. Sadly, just like that, hope had crept back into my life and quickly left. I handed my phone to my mom and walked away.

Please. Please. Don't do this to me, God. I hate you.

I hate you.

I hate me.

I hate insurance.

I hate life.

I hate everything.

I quickly spun into a level of turmoil my family didn't know how to handle. I existed like this for multiple days. I just couldn't cope. I knew my life was over. That was until my mom got a call.

"A program at Kennedy Krieger said they could see you. It's outpatient, and they can treat you over Zoom because of COVID-19," my mom told me with excitement.

I'm in this much pain, and we are dealing with it over Zoom?

"Ok. Sure. Whatever."

We quickly set everything up, and I started the following week. Want to know my mission? It was to prove that Zoom appointments would never work.

• • • ● • ● • • •

AUDREY MARIE

My dear, dear friend. I need to fill you in. I am sure you are thinking, 'Audrey, why would you want to prove that the treatment wouldn't work?' I get it. It seems like an atypical thought process. But when you are in deep depths of pain and disappointment, you learn never to get your hopes up. It is a form of protection. Treatment over Zoom did not feel like it matched the severity of my condition.

What would you do if you felt you needed to defend your condition? How long until you would give up? I'd say I lasted longer than I would've thought.

• • • ● • ● • • •

My day full of appointments began early. I used the basement of my house as my own personal medical space. I threw on a comfy outfit and clicked to sign in for the first appointment. In the blink of an eye, a woman I'll call "Bea" came up on the screen. With her hair in a ponytail, she explained how my appointments would work.

"Let's time how long you can hold both arms up."

Physical therapy was a little easier over Zoom, but it was odd. With each appointment, Bea would talk with me about soccer, theater, her kids, and fall (yes, the season—it is my favorite). It felt like we always had something to talk about. I guess that's all you can do when you get so frustrated at how you can hold your arms up for only four seconds. But no matter what, Bea distracted me. I would get distracted standing because I would be telling Bea about my favorite songs in "Into the Woods." She was always happy and knew exactly what I loved.

I had five minutes between that appointment and the next. This one was with Amena.

Amena was young but incredibly intelligent. It was clear right away that she understood my condition. She quickly explained that I would need a basket full of things that we could use during occupational therapy. I didn't know at that moment that, although OT would be the appointment I would cheat in most, it was also one that would help me manage life most effectively. Both came from the fact that occupational therapy hit on what I viewed to be the most embarrassing part of my condition.

I struggled with brushing my teeth, getting ready, showering, eating, and many other essential aspects of life. That, added to the fact that I had learned not to trust medical professionals, made me incredibly defiant about treatment.

I don't know if Amena knew she would be in for some rough times in my appointments. I didn't. But she quickly earned my trust. From there on, I began to let her see parts of me no one else had seen. I am eternally grateful to her for that, and I believe that is why she was critical in my life at the time.

• • • ● ● • ● • • •

Therapy may be a sensitive topic for many people going through chronic pain. As always, I want to explain my personal beliefs and experience (please know everyone is different). I assumed that if I was forced into therapy, it meant that others thought my illness was all made up in my head. Basically, I was a girl dealing with trauma and just making up this unprovable pain. God knows that was the direct correlation I experienced. That was until I met Dr. Ritza.

• • • ● ● • ● • • •

I jumped from Amena's appointment to Dr. Ritza's, and I have to tell you, I was not happy. Dr. Ritza was my therapist, and words couldn't express how stressed I felt about this form of treatment.

I went into the appointment with the understanding that I would have to defend my pain. I would have to defend that I wasn't crazy (whatever that means). Dr. Ritza started the Zoom, smiling brightly. She was incredibly confident and compassionate at the same time. I could tell she was reading into everything I said, but I didn't think I had to defend my pain. It was odd, hopeful, and yet I was still incredibly cautious. The appointment didn't end well because she asked me something I would never forget.

"Audrey, what if the pain never goes away?"

Is this lady kidding me?

"It's going to." I quickly responded with doubt in my voice as I shifted in my desk chair.

I was absolutely furious. How is that helpful? How does it give me hope? But that's the thing about hope, my friend. It can't be given. Only found.

I also would like to make another point. Dr. Ritza had no desire to tear hope away from me. Instead, she wanted to teach me that it is possible to live life alongside pain. This is an idea I will teach you later, but at that point, putting that idea into my head was the best thing she could have ever done for me. I had never considered life happening while still being in pain. Instead, I assumed the pain had to stop in order for me to start living again. That, I learned, was the biggest lie I ever told myself.

AUDREY MARIE

• • • • ● • ● • • •

I repeated this schedule of appointments for four weeks straight. In that span of time, I learned yoga, got ready every morning with Amena's pointers, and was not having it with Dr. Ritza. I ended up being diagnosed with Post Traumatic Stress Disorder from the post-surgery events that happened when I was 16. I have to be honest with you—at the time, I thought that was ridiculous. There was no way I had PTSD from surgery. People get procedures all the time. And I knew I wasn't weak.

• • • • ● • ● • • •

I'm not so weak that I developed a mental condition from a typical surgery.

I'm sure you are catching on, my friend, that my inner dialogue was not supportive. Although I continuously denied the PTSD, I struggled with parts of the treatment for it.

"Why don't you tell me what happened?" Dr. Ritza asked during treatment.

I began telling the story. By about two minutes in, I paused. All of a sudden, I couldn't speak. Despite my desperate attempt to stop the story, it continued in my head and body. Within a blink of an eye, I was in the moment, yet again.

I suddenly came to when Dr. Ritza started calling my name.

"Audrey, what's your favorite Bishop Briggs song?" Dr. Ritza remembered how I explained she was my favorite singer.

"I don't know." I was in a trance that I could not break free from. My entire body was tense.

"Name any song of hers then."

"*White Flag* is a good one."

I sat in my room as Dr. Ritza played the song. As time went on, I noticed I was brought back to the present. I won't lie and say I didn't recognize this feeling. It had been happening for years. However, this was the first time someone else had noticed it. As I began to do my typical routine of poor self-degradation, Dr. Ritza showed me what my brain couldn't recognize.

Pride.

She was proud of the parts of my trauma I *could* tell (even though my brain made me believe that it was practically nothing). You see, up until this point, no medical professional acted as if what I was doing to combat my pain (emotional or physical) was impressive or even a representation of strength. It's sad, but true. Dr. Ritza's pride was a foreign concept to me.

Not only that, but I was also diagnosed with Functional Neurological Symptom Disorder or FNSD. If you want to know more about FNSD, now may be a good time to flip to the front of this book and read my description of the condition, but it is safe to say I was livid with this diagnosis. That was the most anger I felt towards Dr. Ritza, causing me immediately to lose faith in the Kennedy team as a whole—especially after the initial discussion I had when I was diagnosed.

"Audrey, it is clear your tremors and some other symptoms are from Functional Neurological Symptom Disorder," Dr. Ritza explained in a very sensitive voice.

I'm going to lose it.

"So now you are saying I don't have CRPS?"

Of course, Dr. Ritza denied that, but it was too late. My mind and inner voice were strong. With that single sentence, I had already determined that the medical professionals I thought I had come to trust believed my pain and symptoms were all in my head. I now know this is so far from the truth. But how do you think your mind and body would react after being in excruciating pain and stress for five years? Wouldn't there be changes in how they function?

I also used the fact that treatment was on Zoom to my advantage (or disadvantage, depending on which Audrey you are talking to). During occupational therapy, I would often put my hands out of the camera's view. That way, Amena couldn't see how I was doing the activities we were working on. You see, I did things differently from other people, and I didn't like it—it embarrassed me. I felt this way even, some would argue, especially in front of medical professionals. Amena and I discussed this one day while I was attempting to get ready.

"I would be the last person to judge you."

"I know"

But in my heart, I didn't know. Maybe the second she saw my clawed hands, tremor, and hunched posture, Amena would determine I was faking the whole thing.

• • • ● ● • ● ● • •

My heart breaks for you, Past-Audrey. The system cut you down and ripped your self-confidence apart. I need you to know this. Every second that any individual questioned you has stacked up against you. Yet today, you are standing taller than ever. Sure, it is wonderful and life-changing to be told, "I believe you," but do you want to know something even more life-changing? When you can say to yourself, "I believe me."

• • • ● • ● • • •

The four weeks passed by in the blink of an eye. Although I did try during each appointment, I still kept my guard up. But it didn't matter if it was talk therapy, physical therapy, or occupational therapy, not a single one of the people dedicating their time to me was able to break through.

• • • ● • ● • • •

I want to share something I learned that is absolutely necessary for the ultimate success of any treatment of this caliber. I can tell you firsthand that this is crucial for anyone who is dealing with a chronic health issue. Service providers, family, and even patients *must* see the individual who needs to get better as a whole person. We cannot address only one piece of the body, whether that be mental or physical. Each part that is affected by the condition must be treated. If it isn't, if we ignore any piece, it will get left behind and eventually come out again in another part of life.

Think of people as a puzzle. When constructing a puzzle, we need all the pieces. When we are about to place the final piece and realize it is missing, we realize we still have a task ahead. Because without that last piece, the puzzle cannot ever be complete. Think about letting that puzzle sit unfinished for ten or even 20 years. Will it ever magically complete itself without that final piece?

• • • • ● • ● • • •

I could feel the time ticking away in the virtual program. This was when I had a conversation with Amena, with whom I had quickly become very close and learned to trust.

"As you know, Audrey, we are coming up to the end of your program next week. We will all start to go over your home plan."

I can't do this.

I can't handle this on my own.

I will end up going backward after the only ten steps forward I made.

They are giving up on me.

I guess I will give up on me.

"I guess it stresses me out doing this on my own," I whispered with fear in my voice.

"That is completely normal. We will make sure that you are prepared."

Prepared? Prepared for what? The pain?

I began to meet with each of my team for my final appointments. I was sick the entire day. I had this feeling I could get there; I just needed more time.

"We all know you can do this."

"You have the tools; you know how to apply them."

"You are already doing so much more than you were."

I know each statement was meant to be positive, but they all made me angry. Each final appointment of PT, OT, and therapy reminded me that I, in fact, wasn't ready. And I couldn't do this. I knew I was still hiding my most embarrassing struggles. So many people don't talk about this part of an illness journey—needing help for the bare necessities of taking care of yourself. It cuts someone down, but it doesn't have to. You'll soon learn why.

The following week, I had finally truly given up—this time, more than ever. I felt like I had tried everything. I had finally agreed to inpatient treatment, and it didn't work out. Despite that, they figured out a way to treat me, and I would be graduating soon. Still, I wasn't healed. I remember that feeling—the feeling of hitting rock bottom. Not listening to my family's advice, I refused to send an email to my team. It was too embarrassing, and I didn't want to feel obsessed.

Please, dear friend, read that again.

I didn't want to appear obsessed with my health and well-being.

This was another reaction to the traumatic service providers I had worked with in the past. Although I began trusting this team, I did not do so fully. I was still protecting myself from the disappointment and humiliation I would feel when they did ultimately turn on me, which I felt was inevitable.

• • • • • • • • • •

Sometimes, our traumatic reactions do not fully fit the current situation. However, we cannot blame ourselves. You see, throughout our lifetime, our body holds traumas that we experience. This trauma can be (and often is) placed on us by other people. Medical trauma and malpractice are incredibly real. I am sure, more likely than not, you (who is reading this) have experienced a point when a service provider let you down. You cannot blame your body and brain for protecting and preparing yourself for it to happen again.

· · · ● · ● · · ·

My body and brain began to protect themselves, and I was finally willing to let them decide what I would be doing next: giving up.

Chapter 28

Finding Him

You may not believe this chapter's events. I know Past-Audrey would shut this book and move along. However, I cannot ignore what happened. I believe this was the beginning of and catalyst for my healing journey. So please, friend, hear me out.

• • • • • • • • • •

Two nights after my program ended, my desperation and sadness hit an all-time high. I had felt like Kennedy Krieger was the hospital that could help me, and yet, I still struggled. I noticed that some parts of the treatments were working, but they had yet to click right as the program came to an end.

I reached out to Tia that night. Her YouTube live made me tear up. How could she have so much faith with cancer while I had lost all of mine? Here was the exact message I sent along with her response:

> Hi! So I know this is kind of weird because we literally don't know each other at all. I just wanted to say that I found you on TikTok about a month ago, and I beyond admire your strength. I am dealing with a pretty hard health condition myself (not cancer), and so in no way do I want to complain to you, but you have given me a lot of the strength I need to fight through a treatment I am currently doing. I've been so down, and I look forward to your TikToks and lives every day. I do have a question if you don't mind me asking. How did you get through not being mad at God for this? I'm Catholic, so maybe not your religion, but ever since I got this at 17, I feel angry and almost feel betrayed. Again, thank you so much (and I understand you may not read or respond), but just know you are taking your situation and making a change for others. Only what I aspire to do myself.

Tia responded less than a week later:

> Ah, sis, I'm sorry. I hope you can know that God loves you and he needs his strongest soldiers. I hope you can feel his love. Sending prayers.

It was late at night when I read her response. Tears began to fall down my face before I even had time to realize I was crying. And I did something that I hadn't done for five years.

I set my phone down and slowly stood up. My dog and cat jumped in confusion as to what was going on. I wiped the tears from my face and slowly knelt at my bedside.

"Um, hi God—it's me."

I had no idea what I was doing. It was as if I was talking to a distant stranger.

"I know you haven't heard from me in a while, and I know this whole thing doesn't work if I only pray at my worst."

My breath was shaking, and my eyes began to burn.

"But I really need you right now. I have no more hope. I am suffering and in pain. My life is going to stay the size of my bed."

Tears were soaking my sheet. This time I spoke with God, I made no promises. I made no deals or trade-offs. I simply asked for guidance. Then, I felt something strange.

It was an unexplainable feeling. As I looked around my room, I recognized it was just my dog, cat, and me.

Strange.

I had this feeling that someone else was in the room. A presence I now know was God. He was there. He was listening. And I knew it. I felt it. I felt at peace.

No longer with tears on my face, I slowly stood up. I got on my bed, and I had the most peaceful sleep.

• • • • ● • ● • • •

The next day, I was still constantly thinking about how my life was over. I had lost the battle. My family could clearly tell I was upset and not in the right headspace. They tried to do everything and anything to cheer me up. But no matter what they did, I just couldn't shake the thought that I would suffer for the rest of my life. I felt overwhelmingly defeated.

Despite what I had felt the night before during my brief conversation with God, I figured, yet again, that He wasn't listening—that I wouldn't have any form of divine help. That was until that very night.

Like many moms, my mom occasionally sends me quotes she finds on Facebook or music she thinks I will appreciate. That night, my mom sent me a song: "God's Not Done With You" by Tauren Wells. I barely listened to it. Correction: I didn't listen to it at all. I mean, God wasn't really my best friend by this point. That was until the unthinkable happened.

My sister and best friend, Olivia, came downstairs.

"Did you listen to the song mom sent you?"

Why would I listen to that, and why does she care?

"No," I said while rolling my eyes. "I don't really care to."

"I think you should listen to it. I mean, I know mom does this a lot, but this time, she really might have something," she said with conviction in her voice and honesty in her eyes.

I slowly nodded and went into my bathroom. I sat on the chair I used to do my hair and makeup and brush my teeth, and then I clicked on the link. Very curiously, I pressed play on the YouTube video.

The music video began, and I rolled my eyes. I assumed this would be a "never give up" song, like so many of the ones I heard before. I never used to be a pessimist. I couldn't be since I had spent all day every day trying to make sure my family was happy. At this point in the book, I'd like to make it slightly interactive. We have been friends for a while now, so I want to ask you to look up this song on YouTube and press play. Knowing my story so far, do you see the connections? My thought process as I listened went something like this:

I mean, sure, I feel like I'm at the end, but this could mean anything for anyone.

Okay. Okay. Yes, CRPS fire can feel like flames.

Then, as the title line played, "God's not done with you," just like the week before, tears began to stream down my face. I finally felt heard even though, when I looked up, no one was in my bathroom.

In order to prevent Olivia from seeing my tears, I wiped them and walked into her room.

"Wow. Yeah, that song is relatable."

Olivia laughed. Ask anyone in my family. I hate to admit I was wrong.

"I mean, it's great, but it means nothing. This is my life now."

Within the blink of an eye, I said something that, despite how bad things got, I believed I would never say.

"This is my life now. I might as well stop fighting and accept it."

• • • • • • • • • •

Countless horrific events can happen to us in our lifetime. They can tear us apart and even leave us with nothing but darkness, but I need you to know something. The minute, sorry, let me correct myself; the second we truly decide to concede and stop fighting is the moment the attacker (person, disease, institution, anything) wins.

This isn't what I'm talking about here. I wasn't giving up, but I had finally begun to reach a point of acceptance—of dealing with a reality I'd been given. There is a time to fight against the things that come at us, and there is a time to move forward despite their continued existence.

• • • • • • • • • •

As I laid my head on my pillow that night, I decided to watch YouTube videos. I needed something to take my mind off the idea that I was waving the white flag. As I opened the app, the very first video to watch was: "God's Not Done With You" music video.

Hmm, odd. It didn't recognize that I already watched the video (the app shows if a video was previously viewed).

Refreshed the home page

#1 recommended video: "God's Not Done With You" music video.

refresh

Same thing

refresh

Guess what? Same thing.

My app is messing up.

I clicked the music video and quickly scrolled through to the end. Thinking that now the app would recognize I had already watched the video.

Closed the app *opened the app*

Same. Video.

This whole set of events went on for at least a half hour. I was so confused about what was going on. This video wasn't going away, but the videos under it were changing with every refresh. I had never seen YouTube do this before. I went upstairs to my mom.

"The video won't go away. I don't know what's going on".

In a very calm voice, my mom said, "Maybe you aren't getting what God is trying to tell you."

I can't take this. Where was He this whole time? Now He cares?

I went back into my room and refused to get back on my phone. After hours of staying up, I grabbed my phone and opened YouTube.

Yep, exactly what you think happened.

The video was still there.

I was getting so frustrated. I opened the video and began watching closely. I was willing to try anything to get rid of the song. Only this time, watching and listening was entirely different. I still, to this day, think I finally got the message. It wasn't the individual lyrics or the actual filming style. It was the overall tone of the song. This song said God had started my healing journey, but it wasn't yet over. Despite everything I thought.

The amount of crying I experienced that night was more than I ever had. I couldn't breathe as tears and snot ran down my face.

"Okay. Fine. You get one more try."

• • • • ● • ● • • •

I began the next morning sitting at my computer. I was texting my friend group at the time about the current situation.

"I'm so sorry, Audrey," David replied.

"I know it'll work out the way it's supposed to," Wilson quickly responded.

As much as I loved the whole group, I was getting frustrated by their responses.

Nothing ever works out for me.

I opened my email app directly on my computer. I added Amena, sighed heavily, and began to write. I wrote incredibly fast and poured all my thoughts and emotions into the keyboard. Here are pieces of the email:

> ...I struggle to talk about the harder stuff or what I am thinking, so I am trying an email to make it easier. I am having so much trouble every day lately, and as we have talked about, this is because

I am managing a full day of classes and work. The pain is pretty bad, and I am spending so much time sleeping my day away. It just isn't realistic for what I need to do in everyday life. I need help figuring out how to balance and work with my pain instead of burning myself out and not functioning. You and I started working on that, but since I've seen you, I am hardly eating and I'm trying to figure out what else I can give up. But eventually, I just give up and go to sleep. I almost just said forget it and didn't even brush my teeth for the last two nights.

So, I would like to know if we can do some in-person stuff... I know that if I can just figure out how to function within my limitations, I will be way better off and will last a whole lot longer.

I never do this, so I am taking a shot here. I am even nervous about sending this, but I need to learn to be honest about my situation. If nothing can be done, then we can just keep doing what we are doing.

I need to point something out to you. My entire demeanor changed at this point. In my email, you can sense my determination and willingness to lay everything out on the table. But remember, I had been failed by the medical system repeatedly for years by this point. I was fearful that I would seem obsessive or attention-seeking.

This is such an important concept for you to understand. No matter what you have going on in your life, you are not obsessing if you are unwilling to give up on your mind and body. You aren't seeking attention. Instead, my friend, you are seeking someone to be attentive to you and your situation or condition. Although Past-Audrey had yet to learn this, sending this email was her first step.

Placing faith and trust in Amena and the rest of the team was one of the best things I ever did in my life. It did not take long for her to respond. She explained how proud she was of me for reaching out and that the team would like to put me through to insurance, yet again, to see if I could go to inpatient care.

For the first time in my journey, I was not attempting to prove how treatment wouldn't work in order to protect myself. I saw a glimpse of light in the fiery darkness, and I was willing to follow and hang onto it forever. Sometimes, this is all we as humans need. No matter how dark life appears, we just need to see a sparkle that we can hang onto until it spreads.

Chapter 29

Non-Representative Insurance

A short period of time passed, and I found myself onsite in Baltimore getting tested so data could be sent to insurance. To say I was stressed would be an understatement. I wish I could go back and hold Past-Audrey's hand. The pain and anxiety I was experiencing was unmatched. Why? Well, I was truly giving it my all this time. I was pushing myself to my limit with each test. I wanted to show insurance that despite being in college, I still needed inpatient care.

• • • ● • ● • • •

Let me explain to you exactly where my head was at. I was in a constant struggle with myself and my current condition. I was extremely grateful that my condition was not affecting my ability to go through college courses, however that meant insurance would not give me the physical assistance I needed. I was increasingly frustrated that people who did not understand my condition were deciding my fate. If you ask me? Insurance in the United States relies solely on paperwork and never views the person as a whole. I could never disagree with this system more. Physical impairments should not be measured by mental capacity and success.

• • • ● ● • ● • • •

I returned home incredibly happy and more positive than I had been in a while. The team appeared optimistic about my insurance approving the treatment. I was excited and looking forward to a pain-free life. Let's not forget that despite doing treatment over Zoom, I still believed living pain-free would be the only way I could continue life. I promise you, that would soon change.

A few days of excitement and bliss passed. I then received a call.

"Hi, Audrey. I wanted to let you know that your insurance denied you again. They say despite the statements and reports from your team, they do not see this as necessary."

How does someone continue to fight something unbeatable?

CHRONICALLY UNSTOPPABLE

We live in a world of people who don't believe removing excruciating pain from someone's life is necessary. What a frightening thought.

• • • ● ● • ● ● • • •

I explain this to you, not to make you feel bad for me. I know you care for me already, friend. My suffering is in the past. However, I do want people to be aware of how much our human understanding of invisible conditions, like pain, is lacking.

I was tortured by my own body for several years. I learned how to function to the best of my ability with pain. However, insurance and doctors wouldn't listen, and friends failed to see what happened when I closed a door behind me. They didn't see the tears rush down my face as I held my hands in front of me. They didn't see the pain that caused me to throw up.

You may be able to relate to this. If you can, I would like to tell you to be proud of how you fight to do things in public. But more so, I'm proud of how you fight in private.

• • • ● ● • ● ● • • •

Not long after the call, I received an email. It came from my point of contact for Kennedy Krieger. She said that although insurance denied me once again, my team would like to start the program with me in person.

They weren't giving up on me. I'm not crazy.

I had all the feelings you could possibly imagine.

Fear, relief, excitement, anxiety, there wasn't a single emotion I could select and stay on. But to be honest, it didn't matter. All that mattered was that I could finally breathe and sit back while having others carry the weight of my pain for a few weeks.

Chapter 30

The Fight of My Life

Within a week, I was on my way to Baltimore, Maryland, to fight for my life. There were so many times I felt like I should quit—the trauma after surgery, the CRPS diagnosis, OT and PT not working, a therapist claiming that my CRPS came from my father leaving, new diagnoses—the list goes on and on. And while all this was happening in my life, I was gaining and losing friends constantly. Very few stuck with me the whole way through.

When I walked into the building I would be spending every weekday in for the next two months, I was terrified. Although it didn't look like a hospital, the sounds and smells still caused me stress. Not only this, but the nurse and lead doctors had to do intake, which meant getting measurements and retelling the same story I had relayed for the past several years.

Sure, I was stressed. Who wouldn't be? Only this time, it was slightly different. I was to be treated by a team I already knew and had begun to trust. Up to this point, they hadn't given up on me. That meant something.

Once I finished the intake, I rushed back to my hotel. I couldn't just start right away because I had a very important interview scheduled—an interview to get into the FBI. Listen, friend, this was an interview I had been preparing for. An interview I had been fighting for. And as you'd expect, it was intimidating. Once I finished it, I rushed back to the program. The minute I walked in, I saw Amena standing at the entrance. My stomach immediately fell to the floor.

Breathe. I can do this. This is it.

"Ready, Audrey?" Amena smiled.

I sighed, "I guess."

This was the start of a long and grueling process. The difference now was that I was ready to leave nothing unturned. Okay, okay, there were times that I didn't want to even peak under the stone, let alone flip it over. But I truly felt as if this was my last chance.

• • • • ● • ● • • •

Before I continue to share the next parts of my journey, I must say that the treatment journey for people with chronic pain does not always look the same. However, that is an important part of CRPS treatment: It must be personalized to each individual. Not only this, but you must be in a place in your journey to be fully ready to leave nothing untouched. The openness of trying what your medical team suggests is just as important as getting yourself there. This is how the mindset changes from working *against* the pain to working *with* the pain. I'm here to tell you that that is the key to becoming free from your condition. We can't wait for our bodies to be free from pain to live. We simply can't.

• • • • • • • • • •

Most days of treatment looked the same: I woke up in my hotel, got ready, asked the valet to get my car, went to treatment for four hours, returned to the hotel, and cried.

I struggled with eating due to the pain and a loss of motivation.

On the weekends, I attempted to refresh as family members and friends came to visit. This was still during the COVID-19 lockdowns, which meant that many people were able to work remotely, even while living with me in the hotel. I was blessed that Olivia was there to entertain me when I was struggling the most.

AUDREY MARIE

• • • • ● • ● • • •

Having a community that fully believes someone with chronic pain is critical to the individual in treatment. This may look different for everyone. However, if you know someone going through chronic pain, become a part of their community. Your presence may be life-changing.

• • • • ● • ● • • •

The first two weeks of my treatment were standard and similar to the treatment I received in my own basement. The slight difference? My team gained significant trust from me. I was finding myself excited to go into treatment and show them how well I could do. They pointed out every little improvement.

My friend, understand this: when your outside medical team is proud of every accomplishment (big or small), you may begin to internalize it. For example, I was embarrassed about a task I was asked to do in occupational therapy: picking up blocks and moving them from one side of a box to another. It felt childish and like I shouldn't be doing it as a 21-year-old. However, that task was considered incredible and significant within the medical team.

By the second week, I noticed I was quickly becoming proud of myself for doing the now important tasks that I had thought so little of in the beginning. I didn't discuss every detail with my family, however. Sometimes, it is best to make your world small in order to focus solely on you.

Day in and day out, I did a wide variety of tasks. Treadmill, yoga, stairs, VR headset, baking, the list goes on and on. In each day, it didn't matter how much I got done—it was the fact that every activity caused me immeasurable pain. But by accomplishing them, I showed my body that I was able to live life without causing myself *physical* harm.

• • • • • • • • • •

I want to share with you this mindset. I understand that doing everything that causes pain may sound brutal. However, the reasoning is very specific. When your body is under attack from pain that it cannot understand the cause of, it will potentially make your mind avoidant. The shower that causes pain? Ok, I will shower differently. Stirring the cake batter? No more cakes. After many years, you will realize your list of "cannots" becomes never-ending. The fear of worsening pain overpowers your processing. Things become dangerous to your brain. Part of treatment is showing your body and mind that you can do everything. That there is no worry about physical harm. I can say from experience, eventually the activities become less painful and scary.

• • • ● • ● • • •

My entire team became my cheerleaders. They fought against my brain, telling me to question every aspect of my condition. Along with their cheers came the education they imparted to me. I worked with neuropsychology multiple times a week, learning about CRPS and FNSD.

"How is your understanding of FNSD and CRPS?" the neuropsychologist asked expectantly.

"Fine." Ask any of my medical team. *Fine* was my catchphrase.

The neuropsychologist figured out comparisons that helped me learn. "Think of it like this. Your brain pathways are like a snowy road. Some paths have been plowed; on others, the snow has piled up. So, we need to work on plowing the roads and pathways that are blocked. Some that need plowing are those activities that you no longer do."

One of my most significant snow-covered paths was writing.

"So, we just have to reteach me?"

These comparisons helped and made me feel more typical. I realized that the better I understood my brain, the easier time I had in treatment. My brain stopped fighting against itself. That was until the beginning of week three hit.

I woke up to snow rushing onto the city streets. It was beautiful as I sat at the hotel desk in front of my window. But as I attempted to practice writing, I slammed the marker down.

I can't do this.

It's not working.

I need to just move on from this.

This team will give up on me in a week.

It's made up.

It's all in my brain.

This is in my head.

I'm done.

Despite my racing thoughts, I got ready and headed to treatment. Bea could tell that something was wrong. I didn't care to try hard during the exercises.

"Let's do some yoga today. I feel like you may need to focus on relaxing your body."

Goodness sakes. Let's try to calm down a body screaming for help.

Internally, I realized focusing on the yoga video did bring my focus down. I stopped thinking and started simply following the instructions. Being my friend, let me ask you this: Do you think stubborn Audrey admitted that?

Absolutely not.

Next was Dr. Ritza, and I was not excited. I didn't want her to break through my walls when I was feeling more vulnerable.

"What is going on, Audrey?" Dr. Ritza quickly recognized something was off in our Monday appointment.

"I don't know. I'm just upset." I was trying everything I could not to cry.

"Tell me what's going on."

"I just can tell I'm giving up. This is the point in treatments when I stop trying. You guys have pushed me hard, and now I'm getting scared and uncomfortable. I don't want to do the things that scare me or cause pain." My eyes burned from the puddling of tears ready to flow over like a pond ready to become a waterfall. **"I'm just scared of the pain."**

"Audrey, let's take a moment. Once you finish treatment, what does Future-Audrey look like?"

With a deep breath, I thought of my dreams. I explained that Future-Audrey would be living alone in an apartment. Dr. Ritza asked about everything down to what I would be wearing.

I explained I'd be able to wear my bracelet, tie my shoes, zip up my jeans, and have a pet bunny. I dreamed so much that I began to get excited. But would you like to know what this also gave me?

Motivation. Motivation to walk through the fire.

Chapter 31

No Embarrassment with Amena

I quickly explained to Amena the conversation I had with Dr. Ritza. I had a special relationship with every part of my team, but Amena was someone with whom I felt the deepest amount of trust. This is mostly likely because Amena was an occupational therapist. I worked with her on daily living struggles—the things I was embarrassed by the most. She worked with me on eating, writing, showering, and so much more.

• • • ● • ● • • •

I wish I could tell you why I was so embarrassed I had to relearn these activities.

I've always been someone who cared what people thought. Living with a chronic pain condition that no one knows about is hard. When someone becomes paralyzed, everyone applauds each achievement. When someone is diagnosed with cancer, people understand that the individual needs extra support.

From my experience, being diagnosed with CRPS and FNSD came with a lot of judgment.

When I showed my steering wheel modifications on my most viral TikTok video, hundreds of people commented that I should "just hold" the steering wheel.

When a condition isn't well known or visible, the general public is quicker to judge. Even with my medical team, whom I learned to trust, I remained terrified that they would respond with something I should "just do."

Please, friend, when you find a team that understands you and doesn't question the activities you struggle with, stay with them. I couldn't be more blessed to have found my team.

• • • ● ● • ● • • •

Amena expressed how proud she was of me being honest with Dr. Ritza.

"Audrey, we can see how much you are working towards your healing. The team and I decided we would like to add another two weeks to your treatment," Amena said with excitement in her eyes.

They believe in me. They think I can do this.

"Okay, that gives me even more time to really work."

By week five, I began believing I could live alongside the pain. Something else I realized? The more I did, the less I was tremoring and the less I was noticing high pain spikes. I was finally starting to do it. I was plowing those snowy paths.

I will be honest and tell you that I frequently cried in appointments—mostly in my appointments with Amena. Those were the most difficult, both physically and mentally.

"But this is hurting," I expressed as I attempted to write with an average-size pen.

"I know, Audrey, but just like everything else, it will begin to get easier the more we work on it," Amena quickly explained with reassurance in her face.

I took a deep breath and continued trying. I can't quite express the amount of trust I had in Amena. I had to. I couldn't trust my own brain and body as they continually told me that every activity caused immense pain. So she became my regulator.

I want to share with you something that I learned from Dr. Ritza. There is a difference between causing pain and causing damage. Yes, chronic pain is REAL pain. Please, don't ever deny yourself or others of that. But the question is, is your pain causing physical damage? In my case, the fire was burning, but it wasn't burning anything down.

I used my education and understanding of my conditions throughout the rest of the treatment. That helped me progress in every area—whether walking on the treadmill, doing arm exercises, discussing what happened to me the previous year, eating, writing, or doing so many other activities. I urge you, if you are dealing with a condition, please educate yourself about it. You can then utilize that knowledge to help you understand where it, and you, are going.

Chapter 32

Exciting, Difficult Farewell

The final week of my treatment was emotional for so many reasons. I had made more improvements within those few weeks than in the past few years. But I had no idea I would gain the biggest wins in the last week.

Bea expressed how long I could now hold my hands in the air. With every exercise, she explained how much improvement I'd made since the beginning of treatment. As always, she talked with me about what I would be able to do once I graduated from treatment.

"Maybe even see if there is a soccer league." Bea was always brilliant at talking about my future. I could never completely doubt the plans she made for me because of her confident way of making them sound thoroughly achievable. I realize now how important that was for me.

Going into Dr. Ritza's appointments was difficult in the final week. I needed to discuss life after treatment, even though that was terrifying. I didn't want to picture life once I went home. I didn't know if I could do everything necessary without having my team with me.

• • • • ● • ● • • •

Allow me to normalize this part of any treatment.

So many of my friends reading this book have probably been embarrassed that they were nervous about leaving their medical treatment. Whether inpatient, outpatient, day programs, or any other type of treatment, graduating can be terrifying. Because once we figure out that life is possible in the environment we are in, why would we want to leave?

However, I need you to understand how you got to where you are. Sure, your medical team played a part in your healing journey—including the nurses, doctors, therapists, and even the security guards, assistants, schedulers, and so many others. But, make no mistake, you got to where you are mainly due to you and your own strength.

AUDREY MARIE

Yes, the road ahead may be an uphill climb, and it may be tricky figuring out how to apply all you've learned to your old life, but your success is possible.

How do I know? Because you made it this far. And the anchor necessary for your future success...*is you*.

• • • ● • ● • • •

Dr. Ritza had used a car scenario throughout all of my treatment. She consistently explained that CRPS was in the driver's seat. It was controlling what I did in life. Not attending a friend get-together; the pain could go up. Avoiding cleaning; I'd "pay for it later."

I understood what she meant, but I always believed I couldn't move the pain anywhere from the driver's seat because of how strong it was.

That was, until the final week.

"I am scared to graduate from treatment, but I do think I learned to work with the pain." I couldn't believe what I had just said.

With pride on her face and pure happiness in her eyes, Dr. Ritza told me something I will never forget.

"Audrey, CRPS is not driving anymore. Sure, it is still there. Maybe in the backseat or even the trunk, but it isn't the determining factor."

Words cannot explain how excited I was. It was as if Dr. Ritza had set me free.

The truth is, Dr. Ritza did what Dr. Ritza does and pointed it out. But I was the one who had begun driving. Words cannot express the pure bliss that I could finally decide where I was driving to. I didn't even need to check in with my conditions to make sure I could.

I was finally breathing fresh air that hadn't entered my lungs for over five years.

I accomplished some of my most difficult tasks that final week with Amena's help. She was well aware that I still had things to work on. For example, I hadn't told her I struggled to shower until the beginning of that week. However, I finally felt okay sharing that information with her, no longer fearing that she would judge me.

And, just as with everything else, we tackled the task.

As we overcame each hurdle, we often created a video, which was awkward at the time. But I trusted Amena's process, allowing myself to be recorded as I confirmed to Future-Audrey that

I had won that battle. These videos were memorial trophies, reminding me of what I had overcome—learning to shower while standing up the whole time, opening the microwave, or some other hard-fought victory. And they were so helpful to me in the months following my treatment. When my brain began to doubt my abilities due to the pain, I would watch myself talk about my successes. And hearing Amena say, on video, how impressed she was with me was almost as good as hearing it in person.

My final day of treatment consisted of tears, fear, excitement, happiness, and sadness. It was a bittersweet ending, but I knew the team would be there for me if I ever needed them.

• • • ● • ● • • •

Quick story: The day after I finished my treatment, I went to a tattoo shop and got a specially designed tattoo of an arrow facing toward me with the date January 7th and a cross. Curious of the meaning?

When I was first diagnosed, I had gotten a small arrow on my wrist facing forward. The intent was that it would remind me to keep moving forward. No matter what, I would keep pushing. However, treatment taught me something different. It taught me we don't have to keep pushing forward without blinking.

That's just avoidance. So this time, I turned the arrow around to signify that I also need to stop and look inward—to focus on myself and the healing necessary in my body and mind.

January 7th was the date I began treatment in Baltimore—the day my life changed forever. I had finally found God again. Yes, Tia helped, but my relationship with God had to do only with Him and me. He controlled each situation, showing me that everything happens as He intends.

I didn't get into inpatient care the way it was originally structured because God knew that being in a hotel room for almost two months would allow me to exert and grow in my independence. And He repeatedly gave me the song "God's Not Done With You" because He knew my stubborn self would need to hear it many times before truly *hearing* it.

Those are just two places where God took control, but I know even as you read my story, you will see His sovereignty all throughout.

So now, my arms tell a complete story. Yes, I will keep pushing forward. But I will also pause and look inward as I was taught on that fateful day, trusting God's presence and control. (I also have two other tattoos, but I will save those explanations for when we meet. And you'll realize then that they line up with the four parts of my book.)

AUDREY MARIE

• • • ● • ● • • •

Please don't confuse my improvements with the notion that I have been cured. Even as I write this, I have pain. Day in and day out, I must work on my writing, exercise my hands, practice keeping up with a schedule, and so much more. I have flashbacks during showers and get tremors throughout the day. However, I am freer than I have been in my entire life. To help you understand this, I want to remind you of a conversation I had with Dr. Ritza at the beginning of my treatment journey.

"What if the pain never goes away?"

I now completely understand where that question came from. It was intended to put me in the headspace of working alongside the pain. Now, I no longer feel the need to put my life on hold until the pain fades away. I have to be honest with you, close friend. That is the best thing Dr. Ritza ever did for me. She showed me that living with pain is possible. No one had put that possibility in my head prior to her except:

Claire Wineland
Bailey Vincent
Justin Baldoni
Tia Stokes

Please notice that the people I was drawn to throughout my journey were those who bravely lived with what they had been dealt.

Justin introduced me to so many people who did just that. It turns out I understood the concept of continuing to live despite everything and was inspired by the concept, yet I never believed that could be me.

· · · • ● · ● · · ·

I want you all to know that it doesn't need to take five people telling you for you to begin to understand that living with your condition is possible. I believe God gave you this book for a reason, and at this moment, no matter what you are going through, you can decide to live.

So, when will you start living?

I know. It's not easy. I would be the last person to tell you that it is. You may not be in control of your circumstances, but you do have control over your response. And the minute you tell your brain that what you need to do is possible, it will start to clear the path and make way for YOU to drive your life forward.

Chapter 33

Same Life, Different Me

Returning home after treatment was difficult. I was terrified not knowing if I could manage life on my own. However, my incredible family set up my home to be successful. I committed to maintaining a routine that included three meals, gym workouts, break times (without naps), and the other aspects of life I had learned I could incorporate into each day.

I had also begun to gain a following on TikTok, and I began to recognize my desire to educate and advocate for people with chronic pain, especially those battling CRPS. I even started a blog that got plenty of attention.

With this carefully constructed schedule and my improved relationship with God, I was living a pretty great life. Sure, the pain was there. And some days were better than others. But that didn't matter—I felt passionate about life again. And I decided to continue the process of seeking to be hired by the FBI.

CHRONICALLY UNSTOPPABLE

There are major steps in being hired by the FBI. I cannot explain many of these in great detail. I must tell you, however, that I was wrongfully denied because this organization was uneducated on health conditions. I know, I know. That's a bold statement to make on such a large organization. As always, let me explain.

As you know, I have a condition called Functional Neurological Symptom Disorder. This means that my body reacts in physical ways to stress, which interfered with the FBI's mandatory polygraph test. To keep it short and legal, I will explain it like this: polygraphs require a baseline reading before the real questioning begins. Then, after the baseline is identified, the physical responses to the questions can show that the person being tested is telling the truth or lying.

However, what happens to the test when the person's baseline changes as the nervous system changes? Whether they are telling the truth or lying, the person (aka me) will fail.

I hope you are able to understand what I am getting at.

After finding out that I failed the polygraph, I spoke with several employees of the FBI, including disability resources. I was met only with denial and resistance. No matter the explanation, they provided me with one response:

"We've seen people with autism come in and pass."

I'm sorry, what?

This statement shows the lack of understanding and pure ignorance I often face with my conditions. I offered documentation, discussion, and proof that FNSD can affect the results of a polygraph. It was frustrating, depressing, and upsetting to know that the organization I had always looked up to was not willing to hear me out. That was the first time I was ever discriminated against due to my condition.

When friends ask if I would work for the FBI if they ever changed their policies, I have to answer no. I do not want to work for people who don't care to understand who someone is.

I did receive a conditional job offer from the FBI before I graduated college. But, being aware of my potential, I turned it down. I fought for my life for several years. I think this was truly a time when I began to realize just how much I can bring to the world.

• • • ● ● • ● • • •

Before I figured out my next career plan, I continued with my chronic pain awareness and improving my health. I had made so many connections, which provided incredible opportunities. I was able to get into graduate school, attend a red-carpet event at the Kennedy Center for a show related to Bailey and

Justin, speak privately multiple times with Tia, share my blog with Claire's family, and bring my organization's boxes for the kids at the very treatment center I graduated from. I was also featured in a hospital magazine and had many other remarkable experiences.

I'm not explaining all of this so that you will compare yourself to me. I'm saying this to show you that whatever condition you may have, God has a plan to bring beautiful things to your life. I truly believe that people who suffer from any medical condition develop a deeper understanding of others. Maybe that's because we have to face some of the most challenging parts of life and have had to fight for even our simplest needs.

• • • • ● • ● ● • •

If you are battling any illness or condition, please don't be afraid to express what you went through, and don't neglect to share the wisdom you have gained along the way. Life is difficult, and we can all overcome whatever obstacles are in front of us when we bravely march together, side by side. I continue to talk with the people who inspire me, including the medical team that helped save my life. They all have created a bond with me that I will never forget.

AUDREY MARIE

No matter what you are going through now or have already conquered, recognize that you have the power to show others that living life to its fullest is possible. In my case, that means holding tight to something that took me a long time to learn: Living with pain *is* possible. I will never again let pain, or anything else, stop me from experiencing all God has for me.

PART FOUR
everything clicks

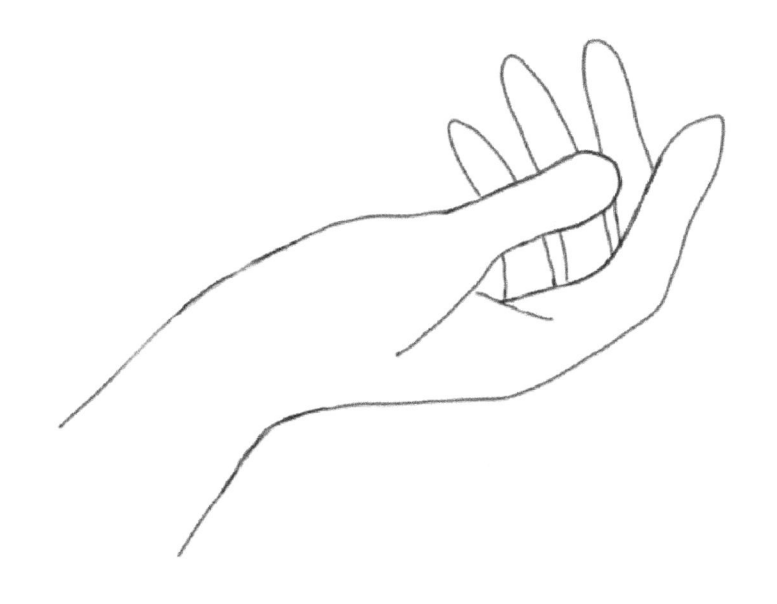

Chapter 34

Right Where I Should Be

Finding a job after college can be difficult for anyone. Most of us have little to no work history in our field of choice and few connections at that point in our lives. It is a recipe for failed interviews. Since I had spent most of my college career building connections only with the FBI, I was stuck with nearly nothing. The only experiences that set me apart were volunteering as a crisis counselor, starting my organization, and overcoming a horrific disease (but that wasn't a resume filler). On top of all this, I had no clue what type of job I wanted. I had been so singularly focused on the FBI that I hadn't considered anything else.

What are some possibilities?

I quickly began scrolling through the typical job sites. So many of the jobs I was interested in, I wasn't qualified for.

Whatever, I will just start putting in applications.

I figured it wouldn't hurt—and what choice did I have? Over the next several months, I went through over 20 initial interviews. Some were with the government, while others were with nonprofits. However, I began to notice a pattern. When asked why I started my organization, I had to share at least bits and pieces of my journey. The moment I began explaining my chronic pain condition, the tone of the conversation changed. At the beginning of the interview journey, I chalked it up to the interviewer not knowing what to say.

I mean, I guess it can be a weird thing. Maybe I should say less.

As each interview passed, I told less and less of my story. I began to separate "working Audrey" with "real-life Audrey." But no matter what, it didn't work.

• • • • • • • • • • •

Listen to me very closely. No matter what you decide to do for your career, know you should not have to separate your true self from your professional life. Employers should choose to hire the whole person for who they are.

Past-Audrey didn't understand that. She was too beaten down at that point in her life, despite her most recent treatment win. Unfortunately for her and most, the few individuals who made her doubt her pain were the ones who continuously replayed in her head.

I'm so sorry, Past-Audrey. Present-Audrey still struggles with that, too.

• • • ● • ● • • •

Day in and day out, I struggled to know my next plan. Although I was in graduate school and educating people online, I still felt I wasn't doing enough.

As you know, due to missing out socially for several years while I was growing up and focused on my health, I felt an overwhelming need to "catch up." But no matter what I did, it seemed as if I could never bridge the gap. And it didn't even help when others told me that they, too, felt socially behind. That's because I had convinced myself that no matter what others said, I would always be more behind than they were. To me, others were behind because they *chose* to do (or not do) something. Whereas I had no choice. Please understand, this is not a right way of thinking. Others may not have had a choice, too. But no one aside from Soph made me feel relaxed.

I needed a purpose. Just as when I was 17 and created my foundation, I needed something that would draw attention away from this horrible feeling. It wasn't long after this realization that I had a conversation I had with Ritza.

"I like being able to be there for people," I explained to Ritza as I told her about Lauren (a 17-year-old girl I supported).

"Audrey. I want to point something out to you. You thrive off of working on yourself so that you can help others. Maybe that is the 'why' you are always asking about." Ritza always knew what made sense to me.

Make sure I am healthy so that I can help others. Hmmm.

Yet again, something clicked. I had the opportunity to be the person for others that I had always needed in my life. I started with Lauren. She had many qualities that reminded me of me when I was diagnosed. I still continue to talk with her and do everything I can to support her. Having someone to relate to is important.

• • • ● • ● • • •

As always, there was a caveat. In sharing my story and supporting those who need it, I have learned that no matter how much someone's story is like yours, they are not you. I recognized myself in Lauren—but that doesn't mean she has my same experiences.

I had to force myself to stop responding to her as if she were Past-Audrey and treat Lauren like the separate person she is. Once I started doing that, Lauren began accepting my advice better.

So, know, if you are reading this, that although someone may have your same condition or life circumstance, each person's experiences and reactions to that experience are unique. That's the beautiful thing about humans. We are all different and special in our own ways.

• • • ● • ● • • •

I was happy with my life, but the fact that I couldn't get a job was bothering me. I knew I wanted to go back to Baltimore and live independently there. The city had become my healing place and brought only positivity and light. Not only this, but I also had the dream apartment.

You see, friend, when I was staying in the hotel, I had a window that faced a building. The building was constructed of beautiful glass and was taller than any other. When I was crying and at my worst, I would look out the window, through the snow, and dream of having an apartment there.

Just as Ritza had instructed me, envisioning my future apartment became part of my motivation. No matter what, I would live there. But the first step was finding a job in Baltimore.

Chapter 35

No Matter What, A Win is a Win

I spent all my free time applying for jobs. I knew my future career would center around helping people, but I was continuously broadening my search. I came to the point that as long as the job would pay me my desired salary, was located in Baltimore, and got me excited for my future, I applied.

• • • • ● • ● • • •

I knew having a job would be tricky for me to figure out. I finally had a schedule that allowed me to be successful. The fear of adding an entirely new 8-hour daily activity was terrifying. But that's the thing about things that scare you, my friend. They force you to grow.

• • • • ● • ● • • •

Scrolling through a job search app, I noticed a nonprofit called the National Trafficking Sheltered Alliance. My eyes quickly passed through the brief description of the organization, and they froze on two words: "*faith-based.*" I hadn't seen any other Christian organizations in the 100s of job openings I scrolled through.

Is this a coincidence? Or is this another thing God is showing me?

From my past, I learned not to question the plan made for me. As I looked at my wrist with a bracelet sent by Tia saying, "Let Go and Let God," I selected the job.

"Referral Program Manager" was the job title. I hadn't learned much about human trafficking in college, but the job pulled me in. The idea of helping survivors of human trafficking throughout the country by finding programs for them to heal got me excited. Not only that, but this nonprofit was based in Baltimore, and the position was partially remote.

Alright, let's see.

I applied for the job and moved about my day. I couldn't get my mind off the potential of the job. It felt right. But, as usual, I quickly began to question myself and my capabilities.

They won't hire me. I shouldn't get my hopes up.

It didn't take long for me to get an official response. Out of pure shock and excitement, I responded almost immediately, which led to setting up a virtual interview.

This was the first job I applied for that I was truly excited about. I felt like it would give me the opportunity to help people directly. You know me well enough by this point to know that's all I ever want. Not only this, but motivation is critical for someone with chronic pain. I knew I would struggle to get up and attend work every day for a job that didn't motivate me.

• • • ● ● • ● ● • • •

The issue of motivation is not specific to only those with chronic pain; however, I'd argue that it is more critical for us. That is one of the lessons I learned from treatment. Placing positive and exciting things throughout our day creates a built-in incentive to get out of bed and is a catalyst to persist through whatever the day holds.

I urge you, my friend, to run to Target or any store of your choice and buy a planner. Each day, write activities you need and want to do. As your day goes on, write down everything you do. This will give you excitement for the day. Trust me. It was one of my key lifesavers.

AUDREY MARIE

• • • • ● • ● • • •

So many things I learned from treatment helped me with this part of my life. However, I want to explain something about my family. During my last week of treatment, each member of my team met with my family. They explained ways to help support me as well as what comments they should avoid. Personally, this was one of the most fundamental pieces of treatment. When your brain is screaming, "Danger!" and "Pain!" you occasionally need those closest to you to encourage you by saying things like:

"You can do hard things."

"You've done this successfully in the past."

"Your past self would be so proud of you."

"You are doing so well and trying so hard."

Most people, including our friends and family, are not natural-born understanders of chronic pain. Just as I had treatment and training in handling pain, people around me also benefitted from instruction. That didn't mean I needed to live dependent on my family forever, but we all need others to help us get through the rough valleys of life. As we hear encouragement from others, we eventually begin to internalize those positive words. Our brains re-learn. Sometimes it just takes time. I agree this isn't the easiest thing to hear, especially for those who are the least patient and feel a staunch need for independence (aka me).

I tell you all this to explain that, as always, my family was incredibly supportive of me getting this virtual job interview. I remember the conversation I had with my mom the day before.

"I don't know if I can do a job, Mom. Like how would I function every day and maintain my physical state?" I contemplated with frustration and fear in my voice.

"I understand where you are coming from. It is typical for a new job to be anxiety-causing. But Audrey, you can do it every day. Think of how much you've been doing."

Ever since childhood, it was easy for me to read my mom. I think part of me wanted to find out if there would be doubt in her voice. That would give my brain all the ammunition it needed to stop me in my tracks, allowing CRPS to take the driver's seat.

· · · · ● · ● · · ·

I recommend that you find positive and encouraging people in your life. Avoid those who may give you the doubt your brain is looking for. For some, it may be family. For others, it may be friends or medical professionals. But no matter who it is, hang on to and treasure them. I guarantee you will need them.

• • • ● • ● • • •

The next day, in my "professional" shirt—and pajama pants—I prepared to log onto the Zoom interview. I wasn't exactly nervous, having done several prior interviews, but this job was different. I spent over two hours reading through the website and looking at exactly what my job would entail. Since this was a Christian organization, I felt like it was a sign. A sign that this was the job for me.

Okay, I can do this.

I breathed deeply and pressed the join button on my laptop.

As soon as my photo popped up, I saw two other women on the screen. They were bright and expressive—unlike many other interviews I had done.

"Hi Audrey! We would like to introduce ourselves. My name is Samantha, and this is Melissa."

They are so kind. What's the catch?

• • • ● • ● • • •

Since life has been difficult for me, I tend to question good things. Believe it or not, I tend to be a pessimist when it comes to the good in humans. I guess trauma can do that to you. It's definitely not a good thing, but it's the truth. I'm not going to lie to you. I can't.

• • • • • • • • • • •

The interview lasted longer than most. Samantha and Melissa went back and forth, asking questions. I was enjoying my time; it didn't feel like an interview. Instead, I was simply explaining the crisis line I worked for prior to treatment and the classes and major assignments I did in college. That was until they asked the question that had affected my outcome every time.

"How did you decide to start your organization?"

My stomach plummeted. How do I avoid my diagnosis and story while telling how I started the organization? The very story that was born from the pain? I instantly began accepting that I wouldn't be hired.

But I cleared my throat, sat up straight, and told them the story. The full story.

That's when I was touched to the point of speechlessness. I looked into the eyes of the women on my computer and saw something I wasn't used to seeing. It wasn't pity or boredom.

Impressed.

They were impressed by me.

I remember both their faces. Melissa thanked me for sharing my story, and Samantha expressed an admiration for my resilience.

For the first time during my job search, I ended an interview with hope and positivity. Not only that, but I had just met two people who made me feel proud of what I had gotten myself through—not embarrassed of it. I have to tell you, this type of person is incredibly rare. Not only professionally but also in everyday life.

By this point in my life, I had begun to trust God more fully. He had shown me multiple times that He was there all along.

· · · · ● · ● · · ·

There comes a time when you need no more proof to trust God's goodness and direction. Instead, you acknowledge the signs He sends in faith, trusting that He is guiding your decisions. It wasn't a coincidence that the organization I applied for,

The National Trafficking Sheltered Alliance, was a faith-based organization. And it wasn't a fluke that the two leaders who interviewed me had not an ounce of judgment.

Sometimes, God just sets you up with the exact people you need when you need them.

• • • ● • ● • • •

Throughout the interview, Samantha and Melissa did not ask me any questions about my physical ability to do the job.

Odd.

I kept wondering when they would get the question of how my condition affects my life and whether I could work full eight-hour days five days a week. Despite my mental preparation, the time never came. Just as my mom and family before, they never doubted me.

People who just met me didn't doubt me.

Again, odd.

What an uncomfortable but incredible experience. Not being asked about my physical capabilities improved my confidence in my abilities. They prevented my CRPS from jumping back into the driver's seat and whispering that I couldn't do it.

Not long after the initial interview, I heard back from Samantha. After completing step two of the process, they invited me to attend an in-person interview over lunch in Baltimore. That was when the fear really kicked in. Fear that could not stay hidden.

I can't do this. I won't.

Despite wanting the job more than anything, I struggled with the embarrassment of the pain-induced awkwardness that is put on display when I am in front of others, especially when I eat.

Maybe they will notice my tremors.

Or my swelling.

Or the exhaustion from eating.

Maybe my pain will be evident.

Or the way I carry myself.

What about the way I hold utensils or use my credit card?

A level of humiliation can accompany chronic pain—an unease that should never be placed on the one suffering from the illness. Despite our circumstances, we should take pride in living life as completely as possible, especially while fighting odds that are against us.

CHRONICALLY UNSTOPPABLE

• • • • ● • ● • • • •

If you are fighting pain or another illness, honor yourself for handling so much more than others can understand. Society, and even medical spaces, often teach us to be embarrassed about our silent battle. Whether by being given slight looks as we perform or receive the explanation of tests or when we are presented with judgmental responses to questions, the majority of chronic pain fighters are taught by the very people we are told to trust that we should be embarrassed and defensive of our condition. I have to say, ask anyone who knows me; I feel enormous guilt for having CRPS. Unusual right?

I'd say disheartening.

Since I wasn't able to assure Past-Audrey, I feel it necessary to say all this to you.

If you feel embarrassed or guilty about your current condition, know I see you. I was, and sometimes still am, you. We have to lift each other up within the community. We know that pain and suffering are nothing to be embarrassed about. We don't choose our struggles in life, and I'm convinced that not a human on this planet would choose chronic pain.

But for those of you afflicted, instead of being embarrassed, be proud of everything you do. You are doing daily life while invisibly on fire. What an accomplishment.

• • • ● ● ● • • • •

After forcing myself to continue fighting for my future, I put on the best dress I had and drove with my mom and Olivia to Maryland. Once we got there, I walked into the restaurant. My future bosses were not there yet, so I went ahead and looked at the menu (my team taught me that this would give me more control). I quickly noticed that they had primarily sandwiches.

Okay, that's a good sign. Sandwiches were easier for me.

I went and sat at my own table. Immediately, I noticed pain in the deepest part of my bones.

I can't do this. Not now.

As I began to stress, I noticed the tremors in my hands and arms increase. Yes, this is partially due to the amount of pain. However, this was also due to my FNSD. The condition worsens with symptoms due to any type of stress.

How would your body react if it was already in "fight or flight"? Would a smaller level of stress still feel like trauma to your body?

Unequivocally yes.

I attempted not to focus on my arms and hands. I began moving them and squeezing my clothing. I also reminded myself that I was safe. Nothing was going to cause increased pain in the sandwich shop. These reminders were helpful...well, sort of.

I continued to look around, waiting for Melissa and Samantha to walk in. As I smiled at a little girl walking by, I turned and saw, coming toward me, the two friendly faces I anticipated, along with an unrecognizable man.

They brought a new person. What if he is judgmental?

I had learned to trust the two women with whom I had shared some of my story, but not the third person.

Okay, okay. I can do this.

As we stood in line to order, Melissa leaned over and asked what I was getting. She was nothing but smiles and came off exactly as in the virtual interview.

We sat down to wait for our food and began the conversation. Samantha explained that the lunch interview was more about getting to know me as a person. I should've been more relieved. But instead, I was more stressed. At the time, my story embarrassed me, and I assumed the more they knew, the less they'd want to hire me.

Yet again, they proved me wrong.

The discussion was going wonderfully. I laughed at something Samantha said as I looked and saw our food coming. My stomach completely dropped.

They are going to think I am incapable.

I'm an adult. I should know how to feed myself physically.

• • • ● • ● • • •

As always, let's discuss this mindset. As you know (unless you skipped some chapters before this one), I had gone through treatment to work on my physical and mental state. But although I knew what steps to take to attempt to adjust my mindset, it was still incredibly difficult to do in the moment. When you live your life struggling for so long, it may take longer than two months to fully make a change and be able to respond to a situation without thinking about it. Be patient and kind to yourself.

Sure, I am telling you this now, friend, but I am also reminding Current and Future-Audrey.

• • • ● • ● • • •

I was eating incredibly slowly. It helped that I was answering a lot of questions and didn't want food in my mouth. Then, Melissa did something that I will never forget. Something I don't think even she knows. She leaned over to me and said:

"Geez, we picked the messiest sandwich. I'm so sorry!"

It was such a simple joke—a joke that had nothing to do with my condition. Yet, it was a statement that gave me an excuse to eat how I wanted/needed to eat. No matter what, they would assume it was messy. A level of confidence washed over me. After telling the stories you have already read in this book, I completed the lunch and went to my car.

"No matter what, that was a win," my mom said with pride in her voice.

"I'm proud of you," Olivia said, looking at me directly.

With tears in my eyes, my heart full, and a smile painted on my face, I simply said, "Want to go to lunch? I didn't get to eat all that much."

Chapter 36

Welcome Home

Within a week, I received an email offering me the job. Celebration filled my house. My family and close friends were incredibly proud of me.

"Audrey is going big time in the city," Wilson said during a Facetime call with us and David. He always knew how to show pride with laughter.

"That is so exciting, Audrey. Working for anti-trafficking is so important." David knew exactly how to point out all the exciting things about a situation.

Countless discussions came from multiple members of my family. This was more than just a new job. This was for everything I had fought for—independence and the ability to move, live alone, and work in a career helping people. I tear up writing this, friend.

• • • ● ● • ● • • •

I'm reminded of a conversation I had with Ritza during treatment. Future-Audrey was someone who had kept me fighting when I wanted to quit. Was everything ending up exactly as I anticipated when I described Future-Audrey? No—I wasn't working for the FBI or wearing certain clothing I had vividly imagined months prior. But those weren't the most essential elements of my success.

Yes, I had pictured every aspect of Future-Audrey's life, but what was most critical were her qualities that had materialized. With her conditions no longer in control, she had won. She was happy and feeling free.

Here is the truth, beloved friend: what our future self owns as clothing or the specifics about their job will never be most important. When you are fighting for your life, that all fades into the background. What matters is that you can lay your head in bed at night, no longer stressing about what the next day will bring—just basking in excitement and peace.

• • • ● ● • ● • • •

The lead-up to moving was incredibly stressful. Every doubt possible passed through my mind each day.

AUDREY MARIE

I can't take care of my own place.

What about making food?

I will start to give up, and no one will know.

I can't internalize the motivation.

However, let's remind ourselves of something. While I might have had more doubt about my overall physical well-being than most, it is normal for all people to question themselves when making a change in their lives. So, while I recognized that some semblance of doubt and fear were natural, I will also tell you I had to fight constantly against my self-defeating thoughts.

Yes, this time, I needed to fight. These potentially damaging thoughts did not need to be worked with.

The time between starting my job and moving went by incredibly fast, but when I met every staff member, I could tell how down-to-earth each one was. One who stuck out the most was Danielle, who rather quickly became my close friend. Melissa and Samantha were incredibly helpful and guided me into my new role.

I'll forever remember getting my first call from a survivor of human trafficking—yes, I was stressed. But one of the most empowering lessons I learned from that day was that I could not only use my crisis line training, but more importantly, I could use my life experience to help others. Please understand—I did not have specific life experience with human trafficking, but I do have experience in trauma, which helps me understand how a caller may think. I was learning how to use my own difficult experiences to help others.

Within two weeks of beginning my job, I was heading off on a plane to Nashville for my first business trip. Let me clarify something—I had never gone on a plane before this. I was nervous trying to figure out how the system of airports works. Traveling had always been a dream, however, so I was ecstatic. This trip taught me many lessons. The biggest of all?

I was capable.

Capable of experiencing life stress and overcoming it.

I don't think my bosses understood the opportunity they gave me. Just as my family and medical team did before, they showed me that they believed in me. Until I could believe in myself, I needed others to do it for me. Occasionally, I still do.

My job and moving made me face my fears of working and living on my own. In my eyes, these were necessary steps I had to take. Friend, as you read this, know I am the most grateful for these events in my life.

AUDREY MARIE

The second I stepped into my apartment, I breathed a sigh of relief. Several times in my short life, I had dreamed of that very moment, and it did not disappoint. I was filled with feelings of independence, pride, excitement of life, and so much more. That moment was more fulfilling than I ever would have thought.

Everything became real the moment the door to my apartment shut as my family walked out. I was alone. I looked out the windows. The single click of the locked door represented the completion of the last part of my life. I saw the last few years flash past my eyes. All the pain, agony, fear, resentment, abandonment, and negativity were suddenly behind that closed door.

Did that mean none of those issues would ever return during my new life? Absolutely not. As much as we wish to move forward protected from the pain of life, that's not realistic. But that didn't mean I would lead my life without passion. On the contrary, I had a burning passion that things could and would get better.

If your difficult chapter just started or is ending, or if you are in a new chapter, know the chapters keep coming. Life *does* get better. I am living proof.

Chapter 37

Catching Up?

Since I moved to Baltimore, my life has been astounding. I have had opportunities I never dreamed possible. I've traveled to multiple states successfully (sometimes dealing with the stress of missed flights on my own). I've presented in front of major leaders within the anti-trafficking field. And I continue to spread awareness and put myself out there on social media. However, that isn't to say I am not doing all this with hiccups. As always, let me tell you a story.

When I first moved, I did so with a mission—to catch up on the life experiences I believed everyone else my age had encountered. Honestly, I still struggle with the idea of accomplishing this feat. However, having a goal like this is dangerous. Experiences are meant to occur throughout life when the person is ready. When they are forced, we risk our physical and mental health. Well, dear friend, my mission put me at risk in multiple ways.

I never drank alcohol when I turned 21. Not only that, but I never went to any college parties. I am the last one to say attending a college party or drinking alcohol is a necessary part of growing up. But, as you know, I struggled with feeling behind. Personally, it bothered me that I never had partying experiences. As you can guess, this is a recipe for disaster.

I went through several months when I partied multiple times a week. As I continued doing so, I noticed that alcohol began becoming detrimental to my motivation to get up for work and my physical health. Sure, I had the stereotypical experiences I originally wanted. But let me tell you this: those experiences didn't work with my lifestyle. I was attempting to fight the pain, just as I used to live prior to treatment.

This gave me a solid reset of my mindset. Due to how sick I felt after weeks of drinking, I was reminded I needed to work *with* the pain. By listening to it, I pulled back the amount I was drinking. I immediately began feeling better.

Yet again, proof to my brain and body that I was listening.

• • • ● • ● • • •

Dating was always a difficult topic for me. Let me edit that statement. Dating *is* always a difficult topic for me. Why? Great question! I never dated until I turned 22. How do we make ourselves available for someone when we aren't even fully there for ourselves?

Many would say it is okay not to date, but that was my problem. I wanted to more than anything; I just knew I couldn't. But that was where I was wrong. I was continuously petrified by dating. Letting someone in meant showing all the struggles and pains I have gone through—the very pains I've written about in this book.

In the words of my closest friends, I self-sabotaged. What a mistake.

By the time I turned 22, I made myself go on a date with a guy I met on Bumble. Despite us being incompatible, I won that day. I showed myself that I could go on a date. Not only that, but some of my worst fears simply didn't materialize.

Maybe he didn't think I was weird.

He didn't notice how I ate or held my hands.

Words can't explain the success I felt in every part of me. However, that is not to say I wasn't forcing myself into stereotypes I still believed.

A whole year passed after that date, and I had not been on another one. I finally decided to go out with a guy I met at a bar. However, he never called it a date. Instead, we were simply going to "hang out".

Maybe this is typical. Maybe I just don't know because I missed out on so much.

I agreed to hang out with him at my place. When we walked into my apartment, he sat on the couch with pure bliss in his eyes.

"Just to be clear. I don't sleep with people," I said rather quickly.

"No worries." It didn't seem to bother him.

Before I go on to explain what happened next, know that everything in my brain was telling me this was a bad idea. I didn't believe his intentions were pure. I almost had to cancel several times because even God was attempting to stop the disaster before it started.

We talked for a while, him on my couch and me at my desk. Then, in the blink of an eye, we were sitting on the couch together, watching a movie. It didn't take long for him to lean over, place an arm around my shoulder, and begin rubbing my arm.

Ow. When is he going to stop?

Light touch hurts both of my arms, but rubbing is the worst of the worst. He continued for most of the movie. My body screamed at me to tell him to stop. I couldn't bear telling him because I'd have to tell him why it hurts to touch an "apparently healthy" arm.

The rest of this story happened rather quickly. I blinked, and I was pushed up against the arm of my couch. His hands were wandering in places I didn't agree to. But not once did I ask him to stop. I know—shocking for a girl who seems outspoken.

There were two reasons why I didn't speak up this time. The first is that his hands were no longer on my arms. This meant I wasn't feeling the razorblade of pain and suffering. My eyes had stopped filling with water, so I didn't have to consistently attempt to dry them before tears fell down my cheeks. The second reason is the most important. I didn't know what was "normal" or "typical."

I know. Such annoying words.

I did not know if my lack of socializing while I was fighting for my life had affected my lack of knowledge of dates. I assumed that feeling up a girl you just met was typical behavior. I went against every being in my bones because of my assumptions. I told myself I wasn't having fun because I was weird—things I'd never say to anyone else.

• • • ● • ● • • •

AUDREY MARIE

I am still recovering after the events of this so-called date. The guy didn't understand body cues. Or maybe he didn't care. Unfortunately for me, my pain and trauma spoke louder than my reasoning.

No matter what you missed in life, stick to your gut. I have so much knowledge about life, and yet I question myself. I want so badly to be everyone else that I am willing to sacrifice everything:

- Getting overly drunk.

- Inviting a stranger to my apartment.

- Walking the streets of Baltimore at 2:00 a.m.

- Taking an edible with alcohol.

I want to make something clear to you. If you are trying to catch up in life or do what everyone else is doing, stop. We fight for our lives in order to do what we want, not what someone else wants for us. I continue to have moments of not being fair to myself. However, now I am aware. My friend, I am more aware than I ever have been.

Now *that* is the first step.

Chapter 38

24/7 Guards

Most of us grow up trusting our bodies. Ear hurts? We acknowledge it and possibly go to the doctor. Maybe we buy cough drops for a sore throat. We might even ice a foot after a sporting event. Our bodies tell us what we need when we need it. Sadly, this is one of my biggest struggles in life.

Not too long ago, I was working from home. I noticed I was more tired and achy than typical. Instead of checking in with my body and assessing the situation, I didn't slow down. That was until my mom told me I looked as if I was sick.

I quickly got up and went into my bathroom to look at myself in the mirror. Listen, I looked incredibly sick. I know it seems odd. How would I look sick but not feel it? This is the way I have learned to live my life—ignoring any and every sign my body sends. I know, I know. Not the healthiest way to live, but that is one mechanism I used to cope with my conditions. This was never a problem for me before I lived alone, as I was often told I was sick before I recognized it myself.

My question for you is: Does the detachment from our body ever *truly* serve us? I'd say, sure, when the pain is at its worst, it's wonderful to dissociate and not feel it. However, the issue is that those who practice this skill often allow it to take over and cause severe consequences.

Cut my leg in water in Florida? Did I notice? Not till someone said I was bleeding.

Tore a ligament in my foot? Assumed it wasn't that bad. But now I stand crooked.

Burn my hand? No clue till I saw the blister.

I could go on and on. Thankfully, I can say I have learned to be purposefully aware of my body. I now know that not being in tune with your body can become extremely dangerous, especially when you live alone. Being fully aware of your body is crucial to taking care of yourself.

I lived with my pain in part by dissociating from my body for over five years. That means five years of needing to experience the worst of the worst pain to be affected by it. When Dr. Ritza asked me if I wanted to be able to respond to less intense pain, I did not need to think.

"Absolutely not. I do not want any more pain added to my life."

However, blocking out pain means running the risk of being injured and not realizing it—a double-edged sword if you ask me. And though I now know that being aware of your body is crucial, the fear I experience when I attempt to live back in my body is excruciating. So I am now very careful about what I do, but that still does not prevent things from happening.

Through this intentional awareness, I have had to renegotiate my relationship with the pain of CRPS, which is so high that it can bring me down to my knees. If I strive to recognize a cut, burn, or ligament tear and then allow myself to feel the full force of CRPS pain, I could potentially be crushed.

This is an ongoing consideration I need to have for the rest of my time spent with CRPS. Sure, it can be frustrating and even concerning, but I try to remember that pain was meant to be my body's way of protecting itself. No matter what now-unnecessary protection your body or mind is giving you, thank it. How amazing is it that your body could discover a way to make you live through something horrible? Now, you just have to teach it, and yourself, when it is safe to put the guard down and when you need to put it up. Trust me, I get it. My guard is thick and difficult to maneuver. It may take me longer to finesse the system, but mark my words, I will succeed.

Chapter 39

Driver's Seat

Here I am—writing this final chapter as I look out of my apartment window at the night sky and city lights. I am in complete shock that I have made it from where I started to where I am now. I am the person I always dreamed of being. That is not to say I have the exact job, relationships, location, and other things I originally wanted. No—my victory hinges on my emergent personality, morals, beliefs, and strength. That is what I dreamed of. These are the most essential elements of a person. They show us who we truly are and guide our transformations throughout life.

Although events and moments fall into place every single day of my life, that's not to say that I am living without difficulties and challenges. To this day, I still struggle with navigating daily life in pain. There are times I doubt myself and my capabilities, and times I want to stay in bed to avoid the pain. I'm not going to tell you that the pain is worth it. You've read through my whole book, so you likely know that I am not someone who will tell you a happily-ever-after story. Instead, my very close friend, let me give you the realities.

Life is hard. Sometimes, the pain can be unbearable. Please read that last sentence again. Some*times,* the pain can be unbearable. Still, I refuse to say 24 hours of pain makes a bad day. Our bodies are constantly shifting and changing based on our environment. There is no point in attempting to predict our future hours or minutes when there are no guarantees of what is to come.

• • • • ● • ● • • •

I don't know if you have heard of the well-known "Spoon Theory." If you haven't, let me explain. The Spoon Theory was developed to explain how a person can handle their chronic illness throughout the day. Each spoon represents strength and energy, so let's say someone started the day with 12 spoons. Every activity or event that occurs takes away one or more spoons.

Brushing teeth? Take away one spoon. Going to the gym? Take away two spoons. Completing a stressful assignment? Take away five spoons. By the time you are out of spoons, you are completely out of energy and cannot do anything else.

I have to be honest with you. I don't like this theory. It's not fair to your brain or body. Here is my adjusted theory.

I believe it is possible to start a day with 12 spoons. However, what the current Spoon Theory misses is the ability to gain spoons back. So, I adhere to an Adjusted Spoon Theory.

Brushing teeth? Take away one spoon. Ten-minute rest? Add one spoon. Going to the gym? Take away two spoons. Meditation, drinking water, and rest? Add four spoons.

By the time your day is over, you may have four spoons left, which then shift to the next day, starting you at 16 spoons. My theory is that we can gain spoons back. Self-care mixed with daily activities helps our body process throughout the day.

• • • ● • ● • • •

Now, I get what you are thinking. Why come up with my own theory and put it in my book? That is the point of all I have poured out to you.

No matter what we are going through, we can develop a mindset that puts us in the driver's seat. My Adjusted Spoon Theory will enable you to work alongside pain. By allowing pain to have the upper hand, we can run out of spoons before our day even ends.

In other words, we work against the pain until the pain takes over. That is the mindset that kept me stuck for so many years.

• • • ● • ● • • •

Navigating life after all I have been through has been challenging. I have been judged, ridiculed, and questioned in my pain. The general public struggles to wrap their brains around intense pain that cannot be seen in any way. And trust me, I've heard it all.

"Why can you go out on a date, but then not hang out with me?"

"What is really going on with why you aren't interested in dating?"

"I see you all happy on social media, but then you say you are struggling in real life."

"Are you sure you can do that, you know, with your pain?"

The judgmental list of statements and questions can run for pages. Every one of these comments has been said to me while I was writing this book. I would be lying to you if I said they didn't hurt. However, I do my best to disregard comments from people who don't understand. Yes, I suffer silently in debilitating pain, stress, and flashbacks. But I suffer while excelling in my job, posting on social media, writing a book, encouraging myself to have new experiences, mentoring those struggling with chronic pain, visiting my nieces and family, and so much more. How cool is it knowing that every activity or event completed is a win?

I am not perfect. I do not claim to have an easy life. I won't say I have solved overcoming chronic pain or struggles in people's lives. The truth is no one can solve this puzzle. The reason is very simple: This journey is different for each person. Human bodies are complicated. Sure, you may be reading this, and your life may have an uncanny resemblance to mine. However, even then, our bodies are not the same. This book is not intended to be a ten-step book to a pain-free life. I do wish it was. Wouldn't life be so much easier?

The only thing I do know is that we *must* learn to work with our pain or conditions. You have read in these very pages that waiting around to live does not work. So, that's it. Today is the day you kick your pain to the backseat. Sure, it may fight you for the wheel here and there; maybe it will even gain control for a little. But know you will always take hold of the wheel again. If the pain must come along—fine. But instead of letting it drive you to your bed, decide to take it to the beach, a performance, work, or anywhere and everywhere that doesn't allow it to cruise your life away.

Finally, please do me one last favor, dear friend. Close this book and put it on your shelf where it can easily be seen. And remind yourself that living with pain *is* possible.

Chapter 40

A Letter from Me to You

There you have it. That's my story of bliss, suffering, hopelessness, hopefulness, strength, empowerment, and persistence. And now, I want to leave you with a letter from me to you. I know what you're thinking: Wasn't this entire book a letter? Well technically. But, now, this is me writing to you from the present.

I'm sitting outside enjoying the beautiful weather with my recently rescued dog looking at me as I prepare to head back to my Baltimore apartment, still struggling not to look back at everything I've been through. I've been through so much. But it all has made me exactly who I am today. So much of my life is going right currently. I still have my apartment and several groups of friends. I'm doing well at work and school, writing a book, and participating in life on so many levels. But that isn't to say that everything is suddenly perfect. Man, oh man, my friend, it is far from perfect.

I still encounter people who make assumptions about me because of CRPS, FNSD, or PTSD. And I still carry so much in my goodie bag from several trauma parties. People don't realize that, but should they have to? Not too long ago, I attempted to enjoy time out at a bar when everyone at the table began sharing far too much advice. They even talked about boundaries and limitations and how I need to set and protect mine. (Now, that's ironic!) The night ended with me explaining significantly more of my trauma than I wanted to.

My advice to you? Live for you. Answer to you. Own your story. People don't need to know why or what is bothering you. It's possible—and would even make the world a better place—if we could all have compassion for each other without being compelled to share or understand all the specifics.

I still struggle with fear daily. I write this with a cyst under my armpit. Almost a full circle, right? All jokes aside, I am terrified. Questions and thoughts run through my head:

What if this stays open?

What if I need surgery?

I can't do this again.

I work.

I have a life.

But I need to tell both you *and* myself: What happened in the past is over. We are different now—we have grown. Our bodies are different, our minds are different, and the people around us are different. Sure, the circumstances we find ourselves in may be similar to what we have already walked through. I know that to be true. But you are not the same person you used to be. You continue to grow with every life experience, which means your wisdom, reactions, and responses evolve, opening your world to more excellent learning and living.

Please know—this book was not intended to be a lecture. I'm certainly not an expert on life with chronic pain, let alone life in general. But I do hope to make use of the lessons I have learned. What's the biggest lesson I learned? It's that living with pain *is* possible.

Once you start fully living, despite the pain, you will notice the rest of the symptoms begin to quiet down. I know, the idea is scary. It is nowhere near easy. It took me seven years to learn this. Actually, I am still learning this.

I hope this book has inspired you. I hope it has inspired you to know that being diagnosed with a condition or experiencing severe trauma does not mean your life is over. You are not only capable of pushing forward, but you are capable of truly living. Let me suggest how.

Work with your condition. Stop fighting against it constantly; that will only wear you out. Instead, work alongside it.

Remove your condition from the driver's seat. Don't let it drive your life choices. Once you take the control back, you will see it shift to the back seat.

Surround yourself with those who validate you. And allow them to inspire you to begin validating yourself.

Recognize that trauma, pain, and suffering can give you a whole different outlook on the world. Use your newfound wisdom to help others.

Embrace religion or faith in anything. It may be all you need to stay standing. Be open to having new experiences and giving a belief your all. No matter what you believe.

Finally, know that your life can and will continue. You are going to have multiple chapters in your story. There will be a before and after of the hardest of times.

I see you. And I see what you're doing to fight every day. I give you permission to sit back and breathe.

Keep this book visible and allow it to remind you forever that living with pain is possible.

Made in the USA
Middletown, DE
30 March 2024